Me Time

Taking Charge of Your Life

Dr Sweeny Johal

Copyright © 2018 by Dr SS Johal

Care has been taken to confirm the accuracy of the information presented to describe generally accepted practices and guidelines. However, the author, editor or publisher are not responsible for errors, omissions or for any consequences from application of the information in this book and make no warranty, express or implied, with respect to the contents of the publication. In view of ongoing research, changes in government regulations, and the constant flow of information, the reader is encouraged to check the up to date guidelines relevant to them. Please consult an appropriately qualified health care professional, such as your family doctor, before making any changes to your diet, lifestyle, fluid intake or exercise regime to ensure that the changes are suitable for you.

First Printing, 2018

ISBN book 978-1-9998040-2-2

ISBN kindle 978-1-9998040-3-9

Editors: Sheena Billett & Loulou Brown

Contents

Preface

Modern-day life can be fast paced and frantic. Worrying about a myriad of things, such as relationships, money, career, studies, family, health, appearance, ageing, and the future – to name but a few – is now the norm. This impacts on health and vitality. It may age a person by a decade beyond his or her chronological age. All too often, the time to rest, recharge and recuperate is dwarfed by the mountain of tasks that need to be done. Tiredness, exhaustion and burnout can easily set in, impacting on every aspect of life. Personal well-being starts to slide down the pecking order as diet, exercise and your other needs are brushed aside.

Poor diets are thought to be the largest contributor to early deaths. Being active and maintaining a normal weight could extend your life by over seven years. There is, however, little education or training given on these most fundamental of needs, and in addition, we are often bombarded with conflicting and confusing messages about what is deemed to be good for us.

You could add quality years to your life by taking some simple steps. There is now a substantial recognised body of evidence that supports a certain approach to life. *Me time* is based on that evidence and approach. It presents ways that have been proven to enhance personal well-being, health and relationships, including the most important relationship: the one you have with yourself. Despite the fast pace and frantic nature of modern life, you can achieve balance, peace and happiness. You can live and enjoy the life you truly want to live.

Me time presents a pragmatic, evidence-based approach to diet, drinking fluids, exercise, relationships and lifestyle that may not only improve the quality of your life, but also extend it by years. *Me time* could not only add years to your life, but life to your years.

Your whole life is built on a foundation that is you;
so why not make that foundation as strong, happy, healthy
and resilient as possible?

Chapter 1

Balance

'A situation in which different elements are equal or in the correct proportions.'[1]

Do you truly have balance in your life? Do you live a life in which all the different components are in the correct proportions, enabling you to remain upright and balanced at all times? It seems that modern-day living has become increasingly out of kilter. People become pulled and stretched in so many different directions that their lives all too often become a frantic dash from one errand to another without a pause for breath. Life can sometimes feel as if you are standing on a street corner on a blistering-hot day pouring out iced drinks for everyone who passes by, but at the end of the day, when you feel thirsty, there is not a drop left for yourself.

As time marches on, the opportunities to rest, reflect and recuperate often seem to dwindle, but the 'to-do' list just seems to multiply. The more frantic life is, the more acute and damaging the imbalance between what drains and what replenishes becomes. Time can easily be consumed by commitments and responsibilities to family, friends, and associates, along with work pressures, not to mention the daily household chores. All too often, the amount of effort required to do everything and please everyone spirals up to a point where a person's own needs, wants and well-being are increasingly ignored. Harmony and balance in life begin to seem like fanciful dreams.

When time becomes increasingly squeezed, the first things to get sacrificed tend to be those that replenish, re-energise and relax. You may start to forget to take care of your own health and needs while trying to please everyone else. A lack of personal downtime and exercise, along with the development of poor eating habits can so easily become the norm; no more *me time*. Despite the external persona portrayed, most people feel under pressure as the pace of modern life seems to quicken and the list of demands constantly grows. It can feel like running on a treadmill with a speed dial that is constantly being turned up.

If this imbalance between what replenishes and what drains remains uncorrected, then chronic fatigue, exhaustion and burnout can easily set in. You may start to feel trapped in a particular life situation, unable to identify any opportunities for change. People often become increasingly unhappy with how things are and begin to imagine an alternative existence; maybe if certain goals had been achieved, or if the people in their lives had behaved differently, things would be so much better now. Although most people can generally cope with limited periods of imbalance in their lives, if there is inadequate *me time* over a prolonged period, inevitably there will come a tipping point where the unrelenting strain of a fast-paced life will start to impact on both their physical and mental health.

It does not have to be this way. There is an achievable harmony and balance in life, regardless of who you are or what your life situation is. Although people may continually make excuses or put obstacles in the way of changing their lives, there is always a choice. There *is* another way!

You can have peace and balance in a world of increasing complexity and chaos. Everyone needs *me time*, regardless of who they are, what they do, what cards life has dealt them, or how important, or not, they think they are. Whoever we are, a burden can only be carried for so long before it starts to weigh too heavily and pull us down.

Me time is crucial for personal growth and it may be surprising to discover ways in which you can achieve it, despite a frantic lifestyle. Everybody has varying sized mountains of 'stuff' to get through, but if you don't take care of yourself, in the long run you are not going to be any good to anybody else as your well-being starts to suffer. Let's face it, modern-day life is hectic! It pulls you in multiple directions with seemingly very little time left for the self. As you try to please everybody else, your needs all too frequently slip to the bottom of the pile.

When you remember your childhood, life seemed so much simpler then. Life was experienced more in the moment, rather than lamenting about the past or obsessively worrying about the future. You did more of the things that you enjoyed and got more out of doing them. Meeting up with friends, socialising, exploring, being curious and trying new things were a given. Teenage years bring their own new experiences, opportunities and challenges. A teenager has to grapple with a changing identity, body and mindset. In addition, an immense amount of pressure may be felt to achieve academically, and he or she is expected to make big life decisions, such as what career to pursue, but even so, there are hopes, plans, aspirations and dreams.

Stepping out into the adult world brings with it a whole new set of opportunities, possibilities, responsibilities and challenges. Fresh experiences come from having a job, the need to budget, to borrow and pay bills as people increasingly stand on their own two feet. Then there may be other challenges, such as children, a demanding career and ageing parents. Multitasking becomes the norm. In trying to push through and complete the 'million-and-one' things that have to be done, you can become so preoccupied with the next tasks you have to do that you stop focusing on what you are actually doing *now*. There seems to be less time for the childlike exploring or curiosity about life, as even a five-minute sit-down or break becomes a life-saver.

As things become more complex and time is increasingly squeezed, *me* seems to fall down the pecking order of priorities. Activities that once sustained you and made you feel good can so easily fall by the wayside. Your passions, plans, aspirations and dreams can easily get brushed to one side. You may end up sacrificing leisure time, hobbies, exercising, healthy eating, social activities and quality time with the people close to you to the detriment of your well-being.

It should not, and does not, have to be this way! No human being can carry on giving constantly without taking proportionate respite to recharge his or her batteries. You cannot be everything for everyone and very little, or nothing, for yourself. It is every human being's fundamental right to have time for him- or herself and enjoy what life has to offer. There needs to be a balance that incorporates healthy eating, exercising, and proportionate downtime, in addition to carrying out your responsibilities to the best of your ability – adequately rested, recharged, and in prime shape to do so.

People need different types of time in their lives: good quality time with their partner, children, relatives and friends is very important, but by far and away the most important is your *me time*. It is not only essential for your personal growth and well-being, but it enables you to support the people who rely on you effectively. And, yes, it can be achieved, despite the demands of a frantic lifestyle!

If you take one thing away from this opening chapter, let it be this! The person with the greatest knowledge of how to create a balance in your life is *you*! Only you can take responsibility and truly make changes to your life. This is not being selfish. If you don't take care of yourself, then how can you carry out your responsibilities to the best of your ability? You will have heard this said before and you probably nodded wisely in agreement, or maybe even said it yourself to other people, but take a moment to really think about this. Can you accept that it is not being selfish to take care of yourself, and to put yourself first sometimes? This can be so difficult to *really* take on board, especially when you have spent your life constantly putting other people first, but it is a crucial first step on the road to regaining balance in your life.

So, where can we go from here? First, avoid putting the responsibility for your happiness in other people's hands. *You* take charge! Only you truly know yourself and can help yourself to live the life you really want. People will continuously keep asking for more from you – that's human nature – so the next step is learning when, and how, to say *no*. This is an important skill to have so that you can start to claim your precious life back and safeguard what you already have to do. Many people find it incredibly difficult to say *no*, fearing that they will upset people or be negatively judged.

Guilt and the fear of being judged are things everyone has experienced and they are often the drivers behind a manic lifestyle. Worry about what other parents at the school gate, your parents, colleagues, friends, partner, and even what your children may be thinking about you, can set in. People may start to become anxious about losing their job, business, home and investments, resulting in financial hardship, even when there is no tangible threat. The mind can unhelpfully start to run away with itself, imagining doom and gloom scenarios that rarely materialise but nonetheless can cause mental and physical strain. Any negative thoughts are best simply acknowledged because they have already arisen, but not compulsively followed or allowed to dominate your thinking, otherwise they will drag you into a downward spiral. Easier said than done, you may say – but you *can* do this!

If you keep taking on extra responsibilities, the things you already have to do will suffer. It is all about balance. No one else is going to sort this out for you; you have to take charge of your own happiness and life. If you constantly take on more and more, you will find there are only so many balls that you can juggle before you start to drop them, one by one. However, at any point in your life you can start to restore balance and harmony when you begin to empower yourself with enough time to eat, sleep, exercise, rest and self-develop. It is essential you do this because your personal happiness and health through the effective use of *me time* is the foundation for a successful life, not only for yourself, but also for everyone else connected to you.

Chapter 2

The Juggler

Everyone is a juggler! Juggling busy domestic duties, work, family and social schedules. There is pressure to deliver more and more, day in and day out, with constant deadlines to meet or somewhere else to dash off to. *Me time* can soon seem like a fanciful flight of ideas. It is as if modern-day life compels a person to be busy doing stuff 24-7.

The internal critical head voice can start to play out: 'You don't have time to sit and relax.' – it's as if sitting down for five minutes for some much-needed respite will result in your whole life tumbling down around you. The internal critic is part of the head voice – the sound element of thoughts that play in the mind like an internal debate or narration about what you still have to do or what is going on in life. Even when you do find some spare time this inner critic can harp on that you cannot afford to relax as there surely must be something you should be doing. Don't believe, follow, or derive a sense of identity from it. The problem is that there is indeed always something to do, but it should *not* be at the sacrifice of the self.

Despite the ever-mounting burden of demands placed on people's shoulders, rather than take some rest, ask for help, or change something, they often feel compelled to carry on from one task to the next. People worry about letting dependants down or being judged as not being able to cope. There may be a fear of being seen as somehow lacking or being ineffective in life while other people may give the impression, albeit superficial, of being able to manage endless demands seamlessly. People often strive to live up to others' expectations rather than live the life they truly want to live.[2]

People try to juggle more and more balls, harder and faster, to keep everything ticking over and everyone happy, often to both the neglect and detriment of their own personal well-being. Negative and unhelpful thought patterns may start to appear in the mind, suggesting that you are undeserving or selfish in spending any time on yourself when you have everyone and everything else to take care of. It is as if the world would collapse if you were not there 24-7.

The harder one tries, and the more life situations one succeeds in juggling, modern-day life can hand over even more to manage. Sometimes people wait in vain for someone to notice the excessive workload and to offer help – but offers of help seldom materialise. As you stand in the blistering-heat on that street corner, pouring out those glasses of iced drinks for everyone that passes by, grey clouds of monotony, irritation, frustration, tiredness and exhaustion can easily start to gather overhead. A constant longing for things to be different can set in.

In the frantic world of today, one of the ways in which to start addressing the fundamental imbalances in life is to begin to gradually carve out some quality time for yourself, as and when opportunities present themselves. While it is important to set aside quality time for family, friends, and your partner, it is crucial that you include yourself in this list as well. It does not matter who people are, or how important they think they are – we all need time to rest, recuperate and self-develop so that we are optimally charged for the daily challenges of modern-day living. It is all a question of balance between what replenishes and what drains.

Draining or replenishing?

If you recall all the things that you undertake in a normal week, how many do you truly do for *yourself*? Make a list of all the things that you have done in the past week and mark them as either 'draining' or 'replenishing'. Is there any balance between what depletes and truly revitalises? Most people will realise that there is a fundamental imbalance between the two, weighted towards the draining. On the whole, they probably give much more than they receive. It is absolutely the right thing to give, as long as you give to yourself as well. Trying to be the eternal super parent, perfect partner and model employee can be draining. In order to survive, many people learn to develop a stiff upper lip and beaming external smile, thus portraying an image of seamless coping, resilience and control.

Everyone has responsibilities, not only to the people in their life who need to be supported, but also to themselves. Individuals can only cope with an unhealthy imbalance in their lives for so long before it starts to cause ill health. In certain countries, such as the US and UK, as many as one in two people will experience a mental illness in their lifetime.[3] Many others may also not be truly happy but fall short of any diagnostic criteria. Often people learn to hide how they truly feel, but this too eventually impacts on their health.

Grabbing something fast and convenient to eat as you motor through life in the fast lane, then clambering into bed late at night exhausted, hoping that tomorrow the pace of life will be ease up, can become the norm. People can become so consumed with the idea of 'making it' and being successful that they can take on too much too quickly and lose sight of what is really important in life. Life is a marathon, not a sprint to burnout.

It may be helpful to remember that you can be wealthy in many ways, such as having good health, quality *me time*, a positive and loving relationship, along with a close family and social network that helps you flourish and brings the best out in you. A healthy work-life balance is also important. Happiness does not correlate with material wealth.[4,5] Unless you start to look after yourself, disorders pertaining to the body and mind will inevitably develop. When that stiff upper lip eventually starts to slip in the absence of *me time*, what will the people who rely on you do then? Start taking charge of your life, health and happiness now! It is your fundamental right to have some quality time to replenish, recuperate, recharge and self-develop.

Replenishing your body and mind

All of us have the right to *me time* so we can not only be in the best place to look after those that depend on us, but also exercise our right to have a fulfilling life as well.[6–8] That includes you too! However, *me time* does not feature in a lot of people's lives at all, or, if it does, the time allocated is inadequate.

Without adequate down time, it is almost a matter of time before you will run out of 'steam'. Unless time is put aside to recharge and restore some balance in life, productivity, relationships and quality of life will start to suffer.[7] All those balls you are trying to keep up in the air start to drop, one by one. It is *not* being selfish. A person is no good to anyone if being overburdened leads to becoming unfit, stressed and unproductive. If the people in your life truly care about you, they will support your right to personal happiness and self-development through sufficient *me time*.

Quality time with your partner, friends and family keeps relationships healthy and vibrant, but the most important time is your personal time. You cannot truly care for others until you truly learn to care for yourself first. You are the most important relationship you will ever have, so why not be gentle, kind, understanding and compassionate about *your* needs?

All healthcare professionals will advise that it is essential to carve out some time to rest, recharge, eat well, sleep and exercise. In the hustle and bustle of modern-day life this seems impossible at times. A person may feel undeserving, think that life is just too busy, or that they don't have time for rest while in the pursuit of material wealth. They may also think that there will be plenty of time for all that stuff in the future, but somehow that *me time* future point never materialises. If you don't look after yourself now, then time is actually what you remove from your life. Stressing, worrying and poor diet can age you excessively – it can wipe years off your lifespan.[9,10–13]

How you look after your body and mind, and develop yourself, not only has a profound influence on the health and well-being that you experience, but also on that of all the other people in your life. The incidence and prevalence of traditionally western medical health problems have been increasing at an alarming rate, not only in the west but also in the east as more people adopt a western lifestyle.[14] It is as if meeting many of our personal needs have been overlooked as technology and civilisation has advanced. Ironically, in an effort to try and make things faster, easier and materially more comfortable, in many ways we have instead made life more complex and challenging for ourselves.

There can be so much confusion and contradiction about what is deemed healthy and what is classified as unhealthy. For example, just surf the internet on something as basic as how much water to drink in a day and you will find different and contradictory advice. For any individual to enjoy life, have good physical and mind-related health, the fundamental elements of nutrition, exercise and balancing respite need to be present in their correct proportions. How the body is treated, what the mind is fed, the robustness of relationships, along with how strenuous daily commitments and obligations are, directly impacts on health and happiness. *Me time* does not just come from small pieces of stolen time for the self, but also from how you interact with every aspect of your life. For example, how you treat associates, colleagues, friends and family, and how in turn they treat you, has an enormous impact on your well-being. People leave large amounts of their life to the autopilot, mentally zoned out, without focusing on how they are engaging with life or conducting their relationships.

One of the most important determinants of the length and quality of your life can be the amount and type of food and drink that is consumed. Most people, however, have had no training on what, or how much, to eat and drink. Studies in the area of nutrition can also be confusing and contradictory. In addition, eating habits learnt in childhood may be automatically and unconsciously carried into adulthood.

As knowledge of the intricate workings of the human body grows, a clearer understanding of the complex, intertwined, synergistic bio-environment that exists within is developing, and how it can be influenced by diet and stress. Dysfunction of this system is linked to many modern-day conditions. These not only include problems with the gut such as irritable bowel syndrome (IBS) and food intolerances, but many other medical conditions including arthritis, skin problems, dementia, cardiovascular disease, liver dysfunction, diabetes, cancer and mental health.[9,15,16] You really can become what you eat.

Although there are actually no such things as 'bad' foods, there are certainly bad diets. A fundamental and key step in fuelling any life change is to first address the quality and quantity of the fuel, the food and fluids, which you place in your body.

Chapter 3

You Are What You Drink!

Having healthy meal choices and exercising regularly could add years to your life, change the structure of your brain, and improves mood.[17–19] As in any aspect of life, there is also a balance to be achieved with the type and quantity of fluids and food consumed.[9]

Although water and food are essential to everyone's continuing survival and well-being, very few people receive any formal advice or education on what constitutes a healthy and balanced diet. Sometimes the information available can be contradictory, confusing, or simply overwhelming.

Research has linked diets that are low in fruit, whole grains, vegetables, but high in red meat and sugar-sweetened beverages, to more early deaths than any other factor. Poor diet has been associated with health problems such as diabetes, high blood pressure, strokes, cancers, and heart attacks.[9,20,21] Most health experts would agree that a balanced approach to both food and fluids is essential to your well-being, but what is a balanced and healthy approach? A good place to start answering this question is to begin with something that we cannot survive without for long – water.

How much water do I need to drink?

This seems like a simple enough question to ask, after all, water is essential to all life. Adequate hydration is important for maintaining both good physical and cognitive function.[22] For a variety of reasons there is, however, no one single amount that will adequately cover every person's requirement. To understand the reasons behind this can give you a good idea of how much you personally need to drink.

First, the total amount of water in the human body varies considerably from person to person, depending on their age, general health, weight and gender.[23] Also, the level of physical activity, as well as environmental and climatic factors alter the amount of water required on a daily basis.

The average water content of the adult human body is approximately 60 per cent of total body weight, but this figure can range from 55 per cent in the elderly to 75 per cent in infants.[23] There is a need to drink fluids regularly to replace the daily losses that occur from your body through urination and defaecation. In addition, there are other losses as a result of sweating and breathing, which are more difficult to keep a track of.

Recommendations for the total adequate daily intake of water can vary depending on where you live and whether the climate is hot or temperate. For example, in the US it is recommended that on average, men drink 3.7 litres per day (l/d), and women 2.7 l/d. In the UK, it is suggested that six to eight, eight-ounce glasses of water should be consumed each day, the so-called '8 x 8' guidance. This works out to roughly three pints of water per day. The evidence base behind this recommendation has been debated, particularly as other fluids should be included in the 8 x 8 suggestion, rather than just being limited to water.[24]

Are all fluids equal?

Fluids such as low calorie soft drinks, weak tea and coffee in addition to water can count towards your daily total intake.[25] The initial concerns over the net dehydrating effect of drinks containing alcohol and caffeine have not been borne out in studies. For example, mild alcoholic beverages, within recommended alcohol limits, may be counted, as the effect of drinking alcohol on increasing urination is transient and does not result in appreciable fluid losses over a 24-hour period.[26] Concerns that caffeine has a dehydrating effect have also not been borne out in studies of regular caffeine consumers.[27] Some of the most common foods and drinks that contain caffeine include tea, chocolate, soft drinks, ice cream, as well as coffee.

Coffee, however, is the most popular caffeine-containing drink worldwide with over two billion cups consumed every day.[28] A daily dose of 400 mg of coffee spread out through the day, which is roughly the amount of caffeine in four cups of average strength brewed coffee, appears to be safe for adults.[29] Drinking a single dose of 200 mg is considered fine for those exercising directly afterwards as caffeine may boost both endurance and high intensity exercise. However, excessive caffeine intake may cause problems such as restlessness, irritability, sleep disturbance, palpitations, anxiety and stomach discomfort.[30,31] Suddenly stopping all caffeine intake may cause withdrawal symptoms, such as headaches, fatigue, irritability and nervousness. Fortunately, these symptoms are usually mild and resolve after a few days, so they are nothing to worry about. A gradual reduction in caffeine intake to within recommended levels should avoid these problems.[32]

Fluids for health

If you repeatedly drink less than your body requires, this may lead to health problems such as urine infections and kidney stones.[33,34] Becoming dehydrated may also result in headaches, tiredness and difficulty in concentrating. Older adults have to be particularly careful as they are less likely to sense the early stages of dehydration. They tend to drink less and take longer to rehydrate.[35]

Children have a higher surface-to-body ratio, so lose relatively more water while perspiring as their bodies try to keep them cool. It is important to make sure that children drink enough, particularly when the weather is hot.[36] Mild to moderate levels of dehydration may impair their performance on tasks involving short-term memory, undertaking calculations, coordination and fine motor skills. Even mild dehydration can result in low mood, tiredness, confusion and anger.[37,38]

One way to avoid these problems is to drink fluids regularly with meals and snacks. The National Academy of Medicine recommends letting thirst be your guide for adequately meeting the need for fluids.[39] Overall, this seems like a sensible approach. The 8 x 8 guidance remains popular because it is easy to remember and jogs the memory to drink fluids regularly.[40]

Thirst remains the best guide to drinking fluids because it is triggered when the concentration of blood rises by less than 2 per cent, whereas most experts would regard dehydration setting in when this figure reaches 5 per cent.[41] Normally the human body is very good at regulating fluid balance – it triggers thirst signals early to prompt drinking. The body finely regulates water balance for healthy adults at rest to stay within 0.2 per cent of body weight over a day.[42] Hence sudden body weight changes provide a good cue that sudden fluid losses or gains have occurred. If thirst signals are repeatedly ignored or not acted on, problems will arise. For example, if fluid losses occur in excess of 5 per cent of total body weight, your body's capacity for work can fall by up to 30 per cent.[43,44]

Drinking extra fluids before and during endurance exercise can be effective in improving performance.[45] However, overindulgence can lead to health problems. For example, acute water toxicity has been occasionally reported owing to the rapid consumption of very large quantities of fluids which exceed the kidney's maximal excretion rate of 0.7 to 1.0 litre per hour. Therefore, there needs to be a balance between meeting the body's need for fluids, and the rate at which fluids are consumed.[46,47]

Sugar and sweeteners

Your need for fluids can be meet by a variety of drinks, including low concentration sugar-flavoured drinks, juices, tea, coffee and mildly alcoholic beverages.[48] If, however, certain types of fluid are taken in excess, they may cause unwanted symptoms. For example, too much sorbitol, an artificial sweetener, may result in diarrhoea. Carbonated (fizzy) drinks can lead to excess wind and bloating.[49] Regular consumption of fizzy drinks may also result in eating more and putting on weight. In addition, carbonated drinks, flavoured water, squashes and juice drinks can contain lots of added sugar and very few nutrients – often referred to as 'empty calories' – so it is best to keep them to a minimum.

Added sugar is a major hidden source of calories that contributes to obesity, diabetes and dental problems.[50,51] To improve health, the World Health Organisation (WHO) suggests that sugar should make up less than 10 per cent of total required energy intake per day, with the recommendation to get this figure down to less than 5 per cent eventually. It is estimated that 5 per cent of total required energy intake averages out to 25 g of sugar per day.[52] Certain drinks such as, for example standard Coca Cola and Pepsi, have the equivalent of about nine teaspoons of sugar per standard sized can. This equates to approximately 35 g of sugar, which alone would take a person over the WHO target limit.[53] However, sugar-free versions of these types of drinks are available and are a healthier choice. It was estimated in 2005 that there were 937 million overweight and 396 million obese people worldwide. If recent trends continue, it is estimated that there will be 2.16 billion overweight and 1.12 billion obese individuals by 2030.[54]

High salt intake has been implicated in stomach cancer, thinning of the bones (osteoporosis), obesity, kidney stones, kidney disease, dementia and fluid retention.[55–57] The UK successfully reduced the average salt intake of its population, and increased consumer awareness following a salt reduction program campaign that was launched by Consensus Action on Salt & Health (CASH). Overall, in the UK there has been about a 30 per cent reduction in the amount of salt added by the food industry to reduce health problems such as high blood pressure and strokes.[58] Following its successful campaign to reduce salt consumption in the UK, in 2014 CASH also launched Action on Sugar, with the aim of slowly reducing sugar intake. A gradual reduction in sugar is proposed so that taste receptors can adjust over time.[53]

It is important to remember that there are alternatives to sugary drinks. For example, drinking milk after exercise and in hot weather may be a better recovery drink than a sports drink.[59] Water, however, remains a healthy and cheap choice for quenching thirst at any time. It has no calories and contains no sugars that can damage teeth. It is also important to be mindful of how fluids are consumed. Rapidly gulping down fluids leads to swallowing excess air, which in turn can cause bloating, belching and indigestion.[60]

Key points for fluids

To sum up: there is no one single fixed daily water volume that will adequately cover every person's need, because what is required varies with age, gender, weight, height, health, physical activity, diet and climate changes. It is important to drink fluids steadily throughout the day, with meals, snacks and around exercise to maintain hydration, both for your physical and mental well-being, and it is sensible to increase fluid intake during hot weather and increased strenuous activity. Most national regulatory bodies will provide a recommendation for their residents to follow. Online adequate fluid daily intake calculators can be useful tools. They give you a more personalised estimate of water requirements after climate, age, sex, weight and activity levels are taken into account. A sensible approach is to take fluids in a controlled, regular and balanced way, but varying intake to match activity, climate and any changes in health. It is better for your health to limit the intake of sugary drinks and not to over-indulge in coffee and alcohol.

As your thirst mechanism is your best guide, don't condition yourself to ignore it. Water is undoubtedly the most important nutrient and the only one whose absence can prove fatal within days. The net positive effects of adequately maintaining your level of hydration on your daily performance, short and long-term health, are quite clear.

Chapter 4

Food Glorious Food

Food is essential to the body, but with the large amount of information out there it can be difficult to work out what, and how much food is in your best interest to eat. Food is frequently the focus around which many social activities and interactions are based. There is no doubt that food can be glorious, but constantly and excessively eating the wrong type of food may have a major impact on your health, well-being and longevity.

On the whole, people love food. Not only does it provide a source of fuel, but it can also be the impetus for family time, socialising, gifts, entertainment, tradition, culture, competition and comfort. The primary purpose of consuming food was originally to survive. Over time, food has generally become more accessible, varied and processed. If you ask people what food means to them, you will get a whole array of answers. The type and quantity of food consumed, however, may either remove, or add, years to your life span, yet people receive little formal advice or training on this most basic of needs. There are many televised culinary programmes, blogs, online recipes, famous chefs and diet fads, and the advice provided on what foods to eat can be overwhelming, confusing and conflicting. So, let's begin with the question of how much we should eat.

Calories for you

There is no getting away from the fact that there needs to be a balance between the quantity of calories eaten and the rate at which the body burns calories. A long-term lack of food will cause health problems. If a person regularly eats surplus to requirement, it will lead to weight gain. However, the body's need for and its ability to burn calories varies widely from person to person.

This variability is primarily down to something referred to as the 'Basal Metabolic Rate' (BMR). Your BMR represents about 55 to 70 per cent of the calories burnt by your body, regardless of what you are doing.[61] The BMR varies according to a person's height, weight, age and gender. This results in some people burning more calories at rest than others because they have relatively more lean muscle mass. Getting older is associated with a progressive decline in BMR; from the age of twenty, this decline generally occurs at a rate of 1–2 per cent for every decade lived, although the variability in this decline between individuals is high.[62,63] As you get older, your declining BMR means that you become more susceptible to becoming overweight, and the days of eating what you want, when you want, without any apparent comeback, inevitably come to an end.

Physical activity is the second largest consumer of energy after BMR. As a general rule, people trying to lose weight need to consume fewer calories than those being burnt through the combination of their BMR and physical activity. To lose weight, dieting alone over the long term tends to be infective, as the body adapts by lowering its metabolic rate, thereby burning less calories than previously.[64] Muscle mass can also be lost during prolonged fasting, thus reducing the BMR further so you burn even less calories at rest. Just cutting down on calories in an effort to achieve a healthy BMI therefore tends to be insufficient; regular exercise is also required.

Any dietary changes are best introduced gradually so that the body can adjust. Sudden and excessive restriction of calories can mess with the body's hunger and fullness mechanisms, which in turn may actually result in eating twice as much food.[65]

Repeatedly overeating even small amounts of food may result in becoming overweight. A habitual energy imbalance of just 50 to 100 Kilocalories per day (kcal/day) is sufficient to cause gradual weight gain. However, even though a person can become overweight relatively easily, modest and sustained changes in lifestyle can mitigate or reverse these gains.[66,67] Before any dietary changes are undertaken, you should consult your doctor or dietician for advice, especially if you have pre-existing health problems, or if you have specific weight and health goals. Dietary changes can still be made, but they may need to be modified to take into account any existing medical conditions.

Calorie counting
Specific advice on calorie intake varies according to where you live. For example, in the UK it is recommended that for a healthy balanced diet, a man should consume on average 2,500 kcal/day, and for a woman around 2,000 kcal/day.[68] Some countries, for example Australia's National Health and Medical

Research Council, recommend no single daily calorie intake value, but instead recommend an appropriate amount for each age and gender group.[69] The tabulated US Department of Agriculture's dietary guidelines are also helpful in identifying how many calories should be consumed for a particular age, gender and physical activity level. Online daily calorie intake calculators allow for the inputting of height, weight, gender, age and level of activity, to provide a more personalised figure for what your daily calorie intake should be.[70]

The different guidelines do agree, however, that there needs to be balance between the quantity and quality of carbohydrates, fats and proteins consumed. There are differences in the nutritional values between food types that may have a major impact on your health. A clearer understanding of these differences can help you make informed choices on what you choose to put inside your body.

How many a day?

Fruit and vegetables provide dietary fibre, which is also referred to as 'roughage' or 'bulk'. The '5 A Day' campaign is based on advice from the WHO, which recommends eating a minimum of 400 g of fruit and vegetables per day to lower the risk of serious health problems such as heart disease, strokes and certain cancers. Significant health benefits have been linked to consuming at least five 80 g portions of fruit and vegetables every day. This refers to five portions of fruit and vegetables in total per day, rather than five portions of each. For children the advice depends on age and activity levels, but as a rough guide, one portion is roughly what fits on to the palm of their hand.

Fruit and vegetables can either be eaten on their own, or cooked in meals such as soups, stews or stir-fries. In addition to providing bulk, fruit and vegetables are a good source of vitamins, minerals and antioxidants.[20] Fibre can also help with dieting by giving the feeling of being fuller for longer. Any changes to fibre intake are best undertaken gradually, as a sudden increase in consumption may cause flatulence, bloating and stomach cramps.[71]

It has been suggested that more than '5 A Day' is even better. 'Go for 2 and 5', for example, is the Australian campaign, which suggests '7 A Day' in total. Australian adults are encouraged to eat at least two portions of fruit and five portions of vegetables each day. Recently, there has even been a suggestion that ten portions of fruit and vegetables in total per day may have even more health benefits. Realistically, however, the vast majority of people find the '5 A Day' target challenging enough and may find talk of '10 A Day' off-putting.[72,73]

Unlike other components of food, such as fats, proteins and carbohydrates that the body breaks down and absorbs, fibre is not digested. Fibre can be divided into two general groups: fibres which dissolve in water, such as oats, barley, peeled vegetables and fruits, or fibres which don't dissolve, which include bran, wholemeal bread, brown rice, and the peel of vegetables and fruits which pass relatively unchanged through the digestive tract.[74]

A diet containing the right type and amount of fibre is not only important for bowel health, but also helps regulate blood sugar levels, and can lower cholesterol.[71] Fibre can help food move through the digestive tract more easily, keep the digestive tract healthy, and prevent digestive problems. However, for those individuals who suffer from bloating, excess wind, constipation, diarrhoea, or have a digestive disorder such as irritable bowel syndrome (IBS), it may be helpful to modify the type and amount of fibre in the diet gradually.[75] The reason behind this is that insoluble fibres pass relatively unchanged into the large bowel, where they can be fermented by the billions of microbes that naturally reside there to form gas which may cause unpleasant symptoms.[49]

For long-standing sufferers of a combination of abdominal pain, bloating, wind, distension, diarrhoea and/or constipation, but with no abnormality found to account for their symptoms, a diagnosis of IBS may be made by their doctor. IBS is a common and troublesome disorder affecting the quality of life of millions of people.[76] Insoluble fibre can sometimes make the condition worse, so gradually increasing the amounts of soluble fibre and reducing insoluble fibre intake may lead to an improvement in symptoms.[77] For example, consuming soluble fibre such as oats and golden linseeds may help to regulate bowel function and reduce bloating.[78] Soluble fibre absorbs water, which helps soften stools and improves their consistency, which is why they can be helpful with constipation. They also contribute to faecal bulk, firming up loose/liquid stools, so can also help with diarrhoea. Many people find that simply taking soluble fibre regularly, will lessen both diarrhoea and constipation related symptoms. Although the effects of changing the amount and type of fibre in your diet may be noticed in a few days, it can sometimes take up to four weeks to notice any benefits.

If you have any concerns about your health, or symptoms such as unintentional or unexplained weight loss, bleeding from the back passage, a family history of bowel or ovarian cancer, unexplained changes in bowel habits to looser and/or more frequent stools for more than three weeks, before attempting to manage any gut-related symptoms via a change in diet, it is important to first rule out any serious underlying medical condition by consulting an appropriately qualified doctor or healthcare professional.

Regular consumption of vegetables, salads, fresh fruit and dried fruit have been associated with a decreased risk of death, with vegetables lowering risk more so than fruit.[15] Fresh is best, but if tinned or canned fruit and vegetables are consumed, it is healthier to stick to those preserved in natural juices or water, rather than those with added sugar or salt. It is better to fill your plate with vegetables than a lot of the other high calorie but poor nutritional-value foods. Instead of thinking in terms of '5 A Day', '7 A Day', or even '10 A Day', as a general guide most people should try concentrating on simply having one additional portion of fruit or vegetables in their diet to start with, and gradually aim to increase their total to the '5 A Day' recommendation first. Generally, eating more foods of plant origin has been linked with multiple health benefits.[79]

Are carbohydrates bad for us?

Carbohydrates often get a bad press, especially when it comes to weight gain, but it is the type and quantity of carbohydrate in the diet that is important. The body can convert certain carbohydrates to sugar (glucose) that can then be used as a source of fuel. The body needs carbohydrates to function well, but some carbohydrates are healthier choices than others. Carbohydrates can be divided into three different groups: sugar, starch and fibre.

The not-so-good carbohydrates tend to be the ones that the body breaks down quickly and easily into glucose. They, in turn, cause spikes in blood sugar concentrations, which are linked to obesity and diabetes. These not-so-good carbohydrates tend to be found in sweets, biscuits, cakes, muffins, table sugar, certain soft drinks and high-sugar containing breakfast cereals.[51] Naturally occurring sources of sugar, termed 'unrefined sugars', such as fruits, vegetables and milk, are considered to be healthier choices; being more resistant to digestion, they don't cause spikes in blood sugar.[80] It is recommended that 45 to 65 per cent of an individual's total daily energy requirement should be derived from carbohydrates. The good carbohydrates should make up 90 per cent, and the not-so-good carbohydrates, simple sugars, limited to only 10 per cent of this amount.[21,81]

Although potatoes are vegetables, they are consumed mainly as part of the starchy carbohydrate component of diet. Potatoes provide fibre, B vitamins and potassium, and have a rightful place in meal plans.[82] It is debatable as to whether potatoes count as part of the '5 A Day' target. Although the WHO and the UK National Health Service Choices organisations recognise the health benefits of potatoes, they advise they should not be counted towards one of the '5 A Day', given their relatively high starch content. This also goes for yams, cassava and plantain. When consuming potatoes, it is better if they are baked or boiled, rather than fried. Many of the health benefits are found by keeping the skin on, so where practically possible, avoid peeling potatoes unless you are prone to excess wind.[83]

Resistant starches can help with any weight loss programme as they are not converted to sugar very quickly. Examples of resistant starches include whole grains, beans, legumes and green bananas. However, in many individuals, resistant starches can cause bloating, excess wind, abdominal cramps and problems with bowel-habit.[49] The way food is prepared can also raise the level of resistant starches. For example, cooking can trigger starch to absorb water and swell, and as it slowly cools, portions of the starch become crystallised into the form that is more resistant to digestion.[84] When consumed, these resistant starches enter the large bowel relatively unchanged, where they can be fermented into gas by the microbes that naturally exist in this area of the body. Food types with which this commonly occurs include potatoes, pasta and rice, which are allowed to cool before being eaten. Reheating these foods does not reverse the process, so if you have a problem consuming resistant starches, it is best to eat these food types when freshly cooked and still warm.

Food intolerance is a common problem affecting up to 20 per cent of people.[85] The most helpful way of knowing if you suffer from a particular food intolerance is to first exclude the suspected food type and see if your symptoms improve. Then, reintroduce the food type and see if your symptoms return. Advice from a dietician or appropriately qualified health practitioner can be of great help.

Back to basics

Before any dietary modifications are made, the first approach a dietician frequently takes is to ask you to keep a food and symptom diary over a period of time, typically one week. Rather than wait until the end of the day, it is best to keep a record as you go through the day writing down everything that is eaten and drunk, no matter how small or large. Note also why you have eaten it and how it made you feel. On doing this, certain patterns may show up, and recommendations can then be made which may resolve any gut-related symptoms before any more complex and restrictive diet changes are suggested. Advice most commonly given to people after this exercise includes:

- eating regularly (usually three meals a day)
- trying not to skips meals or eating late at night
- eating smaller and more regular meals
- not eating fast; taking time to eat
- chewing food carefully and thoroughly
- drinking water regularly to meet your daily need
- limiting fizzy and high sugar drinks
- avoiding rich or spicy foods and those high in saturated fats
- reducing processed meals, unhealthy takeaways, high sugar and salt containing foods
- avoiding unhealthy snacking
- preparing fresh food whenever possible
- lowering alcohol and caffeine intake to the recommended limits

- eating the right balance of vegetables, fruit, healthy fats and proteins

People with acid reflux may also be advised to limit tea, coffee, alcohol and citrus drinks, along with spicy, fatty and large meals. A dietician may also recommend natural ways of helping to improve bowel function. In people with constipation, for example, where the stools become hard or difficult to pass, eating prunes (small dried plums) or ispaghula (psyllium husk) which is dissolved in water before taking, may be suggested to improve stool frequency and consistency.[86] Ispaghula is a type of fibre made from the husks of the Plantago ovata plant's seeds that swells when it comes into contact with the fluid in your gut, resulting in an increase in the volume of stool. The increased faecal mass stimulates the muscles in the walls of your bowel to push the contents of the bowel along, which can help relieve constipation. Unless troubled by acid reflux, peppermint may also be recommended to help reduce any symptoms of abdominal bloating and discomfort by relaxing the muscles of your intestines.[87]

If you still have ongoing gut-related symptoms, a dietician may then suggest and guide you through something referred to as a low FODMAP diet.

FODMAPs

The term FODMAP is an acronym that stands for *Fermentable Oligosaccharides, Disaccharides, Monosaccharides and Polyols*. They are a collection of short chain carbohydrates found in a variety of natural fruits, vegetables and additives. When consumed, high

FODMAP foods can pass through the stomach and small intestine relatively unchanged. They can then be fermented by the naturally occurring large bowel microbes into gas and can also attract water into the large bowel. This may trigger symptoms such as excess wind, bloating, abdominal pain and diarrhoea.[75]

The low FODMAP diet was developed by researchers at Monash University, Australia, along with recommendations on how to trial the diet using helpful advice sheets, diet booklets, and a handy app.[88] The diet works by restricting foods high in FODMAPs and replacing them with low FODMAP alternatives, so that you have some guidance on what you can eat rather than just what to avoid. The diet is trialled for six to eight weeks under the guidance of a dietician. If you have additional medical problems, such as diabetes, this guidance along with advice from your doctor is particularly important. After the trial period there is usually a gradual reintroduction of high FODMAP containing foods, normally one food type a week, to discover which food types may be causing or aggravating your symptoms.[75,89] The next step is the maintenance phase, where you stick to consuming the FODMAPs that don't cause you any problems, as part of a healthy and balanced long-term nutritional plan.

Some of the high FODMAP foods that people most frequently complain about tend to be garlic, onions and lactose. If garlic is a problem, you can try a garlic spray or garlic-infused oil instead. Common onions can potentially be replaced by the green stem of spring onions. Lactose-free diet is a good option if on consuming lactose you experience gut-related symptoms.

Lactose is found in animal milk and products derived from it such as cheese, nougat, whey, butter and casein. Alternative sources of lactose-free milk include soya, almond, coconut, oat, rice and lactose-free cow's milk.

Gluten

Gluten has been a relatively recent introduction into human diets. Gluten is a mixture of two proteins found in grains like wheat, rye, spelt and barley. It gives dough its elastic texture. People who are genetically susceptible to gluten suffer from a condition termed coeliac disease. In people with coeliac disease, the immune system reacts to any gluten containing foods that are eaten, which results in damage of the lining of the small bowel, impairing its ability to absorb food. This only happens on eating gluten.

People with coeliac disease may suffer from problems such as diarrhoea, tiredness, weight loss, anaemia, osteoporosis, skin and neurological problems. In some people, however, it may cause no or very little symptoms, and may be diagnosed because somebody in the family has already been found to have the condition or a screening test was performed. The prevalence of coeliac disease has been estimated to be approximately 0.5 per cent to 1 per cent in different parts of the world. Between 5 to 10 per cent of people do not have coeliac disease but experience similar symptoms to people with coeliac disease on consuming gluten.[49,90,91] This is known as gluten intolerance or non-coeliac gluten sensitivity.

If eating gluten causes you symptoms, your doctor can arrange for blood tests to determine if you have coeliac disease whilst you are still eating a gluten containing diet. Stopping gluten before you have had these tests can give a false negative reading. Once coeliac disease has been ruled out, a trial on a gluten-free diet to see if any gut-related symptoms improve, followed by a period of reintroduction of gluten to see if symptoms reoccur, may be recommended with the help of an appropriately qualified healthcare professional.[91] For those individuals who are otherwise healthy, symptom free, and do not suffer from gluten related conditions such as coeliac disease or non-coeliac gluten sensitivity, there is no need to routinely restrict or stop gluten consumption. Purposely excluding gluten from your diet when you have no underlying health reason to do so, can inadvertently reduce your whole-grain consumption, and may increase your risk of cardiovascular events.[92]

Due to their numerous benefits, healthy choice carbohydrates have a rightful place on your plate when consumed in the correct quantity. Vegetables, fruit, legumes (such as peas, beans and peanuts), and whole grains are deemed healthier choices. However, refined carbohydrates, such as sugar-sweetened beverages, pastries, white bread, white pasta and white rice are not such healthy choices. Simple sugars should if possible be restricted to no more than 25g of sugar per day.[52]

Proteins

Proteins are made up of small units called amino acids, which are essential components of every cell in your body. Amino acids are used to build and repair tissues, make enzymes and hormones, and maintain a strong immune system. Unlike fats and carbohydrates, the body does not store excess protein, and therefore has no reservoir to draw on when it needs amino acids. Therefore, a certain amount of protein should be consumed every day; otherwise the body will start to break down its own muscles, particularly during times of stress.[93]

There are various sources of dietary protein such as beans, pulses, fish, eggs and meat. Consumption of processed meats, such as bacon, hot dogs, luncheon meats, salami and sausages, have been linked to heart attacks, diabetes, strokes and bowel cancer, so are best kept to a minimum.[94,95] For those people who eat meat, it is better to choose lean cuts of meat and avoid meats high in saturated fats. Too much consumption of red meat has been associated with an increased risk of death on account of higher blood cholesterol levels, which in turn can clog blood vessels, leading to heart attacks and strokes.[96] Substitution of red meat with other healthy protein sources has been associated with a lowering of the risk of developing these problems.[97] The American Heart Association recommends limiting calories derived from saturated fats to no more than 6 per cent, so that if the daily calorie requirement for a person is 2,000 Kcal, no more than 120 Kcal (13 grams) should come from saturated fats.

It is also a good idea to consider eating at least two portions of fish every week, unless there is a known allergy to fish products. Although all forms of fish are considered healthy sources of protein, one of these portions should ideally be oily fish, such as salmon or mackerel, because of their relatively higher omega-3 fatty acid content which is considered a good source of fat. These types of fatty acids are vital to the body and brain for optimal function. They have been linked to a lowering of the risk of heart attacks, strokes and death.[98,99] Regularly consuming one or more servings of fish per week has been reported to lower the risk of heart disease by 15 per cent, and helps maintain a healthy brain.[100,101]

Pulses such as beans, peas and lentils are good alternatives to meat as they are lower in saturated fat and high in fibre and protein. For non-meat eaters, appropriately planned vegetarian diets, including total vegetarian or vegan diets, are healthy, nutritionally adequate, and may provide health benefits in the prevention and treatment of certain diseases.[102]

Regularly eating protein can help you lose weight by boosting the secretion of satiety hormones that inhibit hunger, and reducing the secretion of hunger hormones which, in turn, reduces your appetite and calorie intake.[103] For example, if people who normally eat low amounts of protein in their diet, start to get 25 per cent of their total daily calories from protein, they would feel less hungry, be less tempted to snack late at night, and experience less obsessive thoughts about food. Protein is more satiating than both fat and carbohydrates and can help keep weight off. For example in a study, after a successful weight loss programme, obtaining 18 per cent of your daily calories, as opposed to 15 per cent from protein, prevented 50 per cent of the weight going back on.[104] So rather than reaching for a doughnut, a protein-based snack might be a wiser choice.

There has been considerable interest and debate regarding high protein and low carbohydrate diets. They seem to work in the short term, but may cause adverse health problems in the long term, unlike Mediterranean diets which have a relatively consistent evidence base for the health benefits associated with them.[103,105] Mediterranean diets are usually high in fish and plant-based foods such as vegetables, fruit, whole grains, legumes and nuts.

A key issue is the rate at which your body can actually break down, absorb and store amino acids from dietary proteins.[106] The right amount of protein for any one individual depends on many factors, including activity levels, age, muscle mass, physique, goals and their current state of health. The recommended dietary allowance for both men and women is 0.75 grams of protein per kilogram of body weight. According to the United States Department of Agriculture (USDA), the recommended daily intake of protein for most adults who are of an average weight and activity level is 56g daily for men and 46g daily for women.[107]

Muscle building

A number of studies have tried to determine the optimal amount of protein required for muscle gain and have reached different conclusions. Some suggest that consuming over 0.8 to 1g/lb of total body weight has no additional benefit, while others show that intakes of just over 1g/lb times total body weight is best for those training as athletes.[108,109] It is important to eat enough protein if you want to gain or maintain muscle. Most studies suggest that 0.7 to 1g/lb (1.5 to 2.2g/kg) of lean protein is sufficient. As only a certain amount of protein can be absorbed per day by your body, anything above these amounts is unlikely to be of benefit, and long-term excess of protein above requirement can lead to high cholesterol, kidney stones and thinning of the bones (osteoporosis).[103,110] The way to build muscle is through exercise rather than just by consuming protein which is surplus to need and to the body's ability to process it.

Fats

Dietary fats are an essential part of any diet. Fats play a role in the production of hormones, which serve as messengers, controlling and coordinating activities throughout your body. It is generally considered better to reduce unhealthy saturated fats, and instead substitute them with monounsaturated and polyunsaturated fats.[111] Monounsaturated fats are those found in olive oil, rapeseed oil, avocados, almonds, Brazil nuts and peanuts for those without a nut allergy.

There are two main types of polyunsaturated fats: omega-3 and omega-6, which cannot be made by the body, hence their name 'essential fatty acids' (EFAs). It is therefore vital that any diet contains adequate amounts of them. Omega-6 fats are found in vegetable oils such as rapeseed, corn, sunflower and some nuts. Omega-3 fats are found in oily fish such as mackerel, kippers, herring, sardines, salmon and fresh tuna.[68] People who do not, or cannot, eat fish can still get the associated health benefits by getting omega-3 from natural sources such as walnuts, soybeans, canola oil and pumpkin seeds. Essential fatty acids prevent muscle breakdown and help to increase high-density lipoprotein (HDL) levels – which is generally considered to be good cholesterol – as opposed to low-density lipoprotein (LDL).

The idea that you should avoid all fats is a mistaken one as there will be a risk of consuming insufficient amounts of fat-soluble vitamins and essential fatty acids which are important to your well-being; they also help absorb vitamins such as A, D and E. If you struggle with consuming the recommended amount of EFAs, taking supplements such as cold-pressed flaxseed oil can be helpful.

Diet fads tend to work in the short term, but what is required is a long-term approach that encompasses a balanced nutritional plan with gradual and sustainable changes. Your body needs a modest amount of protein to function well, but extra protein does not give you extra strength; that is built up through strength training. Regularly eating more protein than the body can handle may cause problems in the long run. It is best to avoid processed foods and meats high in saturated fatty acids. If there is no allergy to fish products, consuming one to two portions of fish a week has been linked to good health.

The forgotten organ

Your bowel is host to billions of microbes. There are over 1,000 different species of microbes that can inhabit the human large bowel, with each person hosting approximately 160 species.[112,113] This colonisation is referred to as 'the microbiota'. Getting older, the food you consume, ill health and taking antibiotics, can strongly influence the make-up of your personal microbiota. This microbiota plays a major role in health and illness. It has been referred to as the 'forgotten organ'.[114]

An imbalance in these microbes has been implicated in autoimmune and allergic conditions, obesity, inflammatory bowel disease (IBD) and diabetes.[16] Probiotics may be helpful in restoring the natural balance of these microbes when they have been disrupted by illness or antibiotics. Probiotics are considered to be generally well tolerated in the presence of a normal immune system. Certain strains of probiotics such as *bifidobacterium* and *lactobacillus* may be helpful with bloating and flatulence.[115] Although many products masquerade as probiotics, only those that contain live organisms and have been shown to confer health benefits should be considered. The National Institute for Health and Care Excellence (NICE) suggests taking probiotics for at least four weeks to find out if they are helpful in improving any gut-related symptoms, but then stopping taking them if there has been no improvement.

Taking vitamin supplements

Most people get enough vitamins by eating a varied and balanced diet, so extra supplementation is *not* routinely required. There is limited evidence of any benefit from taking extra vitamins and minerals for the prevention of cancer, strokes or heart problems.[116] Taking too much of anything, including vitamins and minerals, may cause problems. Supplements should only be taken to treat any identified underlying vitamin deficiencies, or by people who, on account of health reasons, are particularly susceptible to developing a deficiency.

Vitamin D is the exception, as only small amounts are obtained through diet. Most of this vitamin is made when your skin is exposed to sunlight. Pregnant women, people aged over sixty-five, and individuals with dark skin should take vitamin D routinely. Women trying to conceive and those in the first twelve weeks of pregnancy should also take folic acid. It is recommended that all children aged six months to five years should be given a supplement containing vitamins A, C and D.[68,78] If, however, you do not fall into one of these categories, are well and have a balanced nutritional diet, extra vitamin supplements are not routinely required.

Smoking

Smoking leads to premature death. There are many ways to quit smoking. If you value your health, this one intervention will make a big difference to the quality and longevity of your life.[117,118] In developed countries, it is estimated that tobacco is responsible for 24 per cent of all male deaths and 7 per cent of all female deaths. For some Central and Eastern European countries, these figures rise to over 40 per cent in men, and in the US, it is 17 per cent for women. The average decreased lifespan of smokers when compared to non-smokers is about nine years.[119] Approximately 500 million individuals alive today can expect to be killed by tobacco.

For most smokers, quitting can be a challenging process, and many smokers have several attempts at quitting before they succeed, but this is something that can definitely be achieved with perseverance and determination. A local 'Stop Smoking' service can offer invaluable help and advice.

Think positively, set goals, and a stop date. Consider using nicotine replacement therapies and chewing on sugarless gum, fruit or raw vegetables to keep your mouth occupied. Going for a walk after dinner instead of having a cigarette can help break habits. For smokers, breaking the addiction to nicotine is the single most important step they can take to safeguard themselves and their family.

Take away message

There are no such things as 'good' or 'bad' foods: just good and bad diets. Eating the right balance of lean proteins, fruit, vegetables, healthy fats, along with maintaining hydration, are essential to the well-being of your body and mind. Fresh food is best. It is better to keep the consumption of processed foods, saturated fats, added salt and sugar to a minimum. Your life could be extended by many good quality years by eating a balanced diet that the body requires, rather than feeding the mind empty calorie snacks. Not only what, but how you eat is also very important.

Chapter 5

Fast Food and Faster Eating

With the hectic pace of modern-day living, it is common to grab and gobble food between meetings, lessons, or while rushing from one errand to another. Eating food too quickly can cause problems such as bloating, excess wind and indigestion, on account of the increased amount of air that is swallowed.[120] In addition, people who speed-eat are twice as likely to be overweight than slow eaters. If you eat until you are full, in addition to eating rapidly, you are over three times more likely to be overweight.[121]

Why? Because rapidly eating and drinking does not give your brain time to catch up with what is being placed in your stomach. When the stomach is empty, a hormone called ghrelin is secreted, initiating the feeling of hunger.[65] When the stomach stretches, ghrelin secretion stops and another hormone called leptin is released, which puts the brakes on eating. It takes about twenty minutes after the start of eating for these changes to begin to occur and the message to stop eating to reach the brain.[122,123] Put simply, eat too quickly, and you are likely to overfill your stomach because the 'stop eating' signal has not been registered.

Eating behaviours tend to evolve during the early years of life. Children learn what, when, and how to eat by observing how others behave when they eat. Many people develop fast eating habits as children, desperate to get away from the dinner table, or, if the food was pooled in the middle of the table, scrambling to get at and eat their share.[124] These are one of the many conditioned habits that can be unconsciously carried into adulthood. Like many other daily activities, eating is also frequently done on autopilot.

Learning how to eat more slowly and undoing this automated learnt behaviour can take some time and practice. For example, putting the fork or spoon down between bites, eating more slowly by chewing food longer, and enjoying what is already in the mouth before consuming the next mouthful, can be helpful. A quiet atmosphere without the television on or any other distraction may also help a person to eat more slowly. Focusing on the aroma, texture and taste of food, along with carefully chewing, tasting and savouring the process, may slow eating habits down and help you enjoy and appreciate what you have worked so hard to put on the table. Why unconsciously fast forward through the best part?

It is when people are lost in thought, without paying attention to what they are actually doing *now*, that problems tend to arise. Mindfully eating can reduce both the intake of snacks between meals in addition to overeating.[125] Ensure that whenever possible, under the stresses and strains of modern-day living, that you try to eat as *consciously* as possible – thinking not only about what your body actually needs, but also about how the food is being consumed.

Comfort eating

During periods of stress, the body's fight or flight mechanism kicks in as the mind thinks it is in danger. This can generate the desire to eat food, in particular high sugar foods, as they can be easily converted into energy to help with any fight or flight response. For example, while watching a horror movie, you are more likely to eat snacks that are high in sugar. It is the same with reliving unpleasant memories. A person can easily end up overeating when stressed. It is called comfort eating, but in physiological terms it is the switching-on of the body's response mechanism to danger. The body cannot differentiate between real and perceived danger, so watching a scary movie or recalling unpleasant life experiences can set off the stress response and lead to overeating.[126,127] If frequent stressful thoughts or life situations occur, this can lead to the repeated consumption of unhealthy foods in excess amounts. These extra calories can lead to excess weight gain and its associated medical problems. However, some people may have the opposite problem: when their mood is low or they are stressed, they forget to eat, lose their appetite, or start to make a habit of skipping meals.

Many people go through periods of stress and its associated unhealthy eating patterns, but as the stress-inducing life event subsides, the fight or flight response system switches off, and a more balanced eating regime usually resumes. For some individuals, because they continue to experience stress, this does not happen. They may end up suffering from an eating disorder.[128] Binge eating can occur when food is used as a comfort blanket and an outlet for emotions. At any time, an individual can make the decision to change their eating patterns and stop using food to fix their problems. Mind-based therapies can be helpful. For example, 86 per cent of people who experience binge or emotional eating can be helped by mindfulness-based cognitive therapy (MBCT).[129]

Food is frequently consumed automatically, with little conscious input into how, or why, it is being eaten. Bringing your attention to what, and how, you are eating can also make you more mindful in other areas of your life. It is your ability to concentrate on the small things that has been shown to increase your ability to focus on the bigger and more demanding of life's tasks.[130,131]

Enjoying your food

Increasing awareness and offering nutritional education alone can be ineffective in changing automatic eating habits.[132] Mindful eating can increase the enjoyment of commonly pleasurable food such as chocolate, as well as food which has more mixed associations such as raisins. It can also reduce the tendency to gorge on food.[133]

To truly notice what and how you eat may not only enable you to develop an appreciation for food, but also allow you to obtain enjoyment from other activities in your life that were previously left to the autopilot. Whenever food is consumed, it can be really helpful to be mindful of why, and how, you are eating. Always think about whether your body actually *needs* the food being consumed or whether your mind is using it as a comfort blanket. Occasional treats are not the problem;

repeated consumption of empty calories is. Food can be enjoyed at any time when it is no longer left to the autopilot.

The simple exercise below can help you reconnect with the pleasure of eating food, rather than simply consuming it as fuel as you rush on to something seemingly more important. You can use any food as practice material: a small piece of fruit, a raisin or a chocolate square tend to be popular choices. It is best to approach the food as if you have never seen or experienced eating it before, with an open mind and an air of curiosity. Use your senses of smell, touch, hearing, sight and taste to reconnect with what you are doing *right now* as you eat, rather than mentally wandering off to worries about the future or reliving the past. When you are ready:

- hold the piece of food on the palm of your hand
- notice its size, colour, weight and shape
- explore the texture with your fingertips: its softness and its contours
- notice any aroma as it rests on the palm of your hand
- carefully take the food and watch as you gradually move it towards your mouth, feeling the movement of your arm, along with the natural weight of your body
- gently place the food on your tongue without biting or chewing
- see if you can just let the food nestle on the tongue for about twenty seconds
- follow any flavours being released as they run over your tongue, down your food pipe and into your stomach

- when you are ready, take a conscious bite and listen for any sounds made
- slowly start to chew and feel any sensations that arise in the mouth
- when ready, swallow the food and see if you can follow it as it gradually passes into your stomach
- is there any after taste?
- savour the moment before you eat the next portion

It is not just the consumption of food but the process of preparing food that can also act as a way of reconnecting to what is actually happening in your life *right now*, rather than being mentally absent. For example, next time you make a cup of tea, look and listen as you put water into the kettle or saucepan. Watch as it gently boils and listen out for any sounds made, or movement of the water. Carefully place a tea bag in a cup and observe the water being poured in. Watch as the tea bag gradually changes the colour of the water; savour any essence that is being released. Drinking the tea mindfully is a practice all of its own, similar to the food-eating exercise above.

There is no reason why a particular time of day could not be set aside for this practice – something to look forward to. It can be helpful when consuming food or drink to eat at least the first and last few portions mindfully. If you can do this for the whole meal, even better. Take five minutes, give yourself some time out, and have a break. Consuming food and water is something that everyone has to do to survive, so why not start enjoying it rather than leaving it to the autopilot?

On the surface, exercises such as the one above may appear to be trivial or simple, but they can achieve deep and profound changes in your life. For example, if you cannot focus on the little things, research has shown that you will tend to struggle with the larger, more complex aspects of life where you really do need to focus and concentrate.[130,131] Also, the amount of mind-wandering away from what is happening *now* correlates directly with the degree of unhappiness or stress you experience.[134] If you can't concentrate on something as simple as eating one piece of food, then the quality of all you undertake may be negatively affected. It means that your mind is easily distracted, including when it comes to your relationships, work and studies. Sitting down for five minutes and enjoying some *me time* may also be difficult if you don't train yourself to become *present* in the *now* and hence maximise the benefit of any down time.

Eating that piece of fruit, raisin or chocolate mindfully can be rolled out to anything you undertake in life, with profound benefits to your well-being. Mastering a simple exercise such as mindfully eating one piece of food can be the catalyst for so much more. You can approach any aspect of your life just as if you were eating that piece of fruit, raisin or chocolate, whether that be brushing your teeth, washing, getting dressed, driving, walking or exercising.

Chapter 6

Physical Activity

Exercise can have a positive impact on not only your well-being, but also on your longevity. Surprisingly, perhaps, you don't need to spend every minute of every day in the gym to see the benefits associated with exercising. An average of just eleven minutes of exercise a day could translate into years of extra good-quality life. Research has demonstrated that those individuals who take part in physical activity at the recommended level of 75 minutes per week (min/wk) of vigorous exercise, or 150 min/wk of moderate exercise in total, could add 3.4 years to their lifespan, and at twice this recommended level of exercise, just over 4 years.[135] Vigorous physical exercise includes running, aerobics and cycling fast, while activities such as brisk walking, hiking and pushing a lawn mower fall into the moderate physical exercise group.

A sedentary lifestyle is associated with an increased risk of health problems that include diabetes, strokes and heart attacks. Being sedentary can potentially wipe years off your life. It is estimated that every year over five million deaths per year worldwide are attributable to inactivity.[136] Modern-day living can involve large amounts of inactivity: while at work, driving, or watching television. Time is also increasingly spent on devices such as phones, computers, tablets or game consoles, often referred to as 'screen time'. Excessive screen time has been linked with poor physical and mental health.[137]

Small changes, big gains

If inactivity levels were reduced by just 10 per cent, more than 533,000 deaths could be prevented every year, and a reduction of 25 per cent could prevent more than 1.3 million deaths per year.[136] The increased health risks associated with being inactive were originally thought to be associated with being overweight, but we now know that even if you are not overweight, being very inactive can still reduce your lifespan by years.[138]

Being active along with maintaining a body mass index (BMI) in the normal range, is best for health. It is associated with living just over seven years longer, when compared with being both inactive and overweight.[135] Research into current levels of sedentary behaviour is limited, but it seems that adults of working age, for example, in England are physically inactive for about 9.5 hours per day (h/d).[138] This does not take into account the time spent sleeping. Long periods of inactivity are also linked to low mood and depression, although it can be difficult to separate cause from effect.

As well as maintaining mental and physical health, physical activity can preserve brain size, improve cognition, and reduce the risk of developing conditions such as heart disease, high blood pressure, diabetes and strokes, as well as colon and breast cancer.[19,139] Exercise is also associated with a better working memory in children.[140]

In addition, physical activity can provide an opportunity for both social interaction and *me time*. It can involve the learning of new information such as exercise routines, which in itself can lead to cognitive benefits. Learning to dance, for example, ticks all of these boxes, and is especially beneficial as it is a social activity and can be great fun.

Any kind of exercise can also both protect against developing depression, as well as being beneficial in alleviating existing symptoms of depression.[141]

HIIT the mark

Physical activity can either be performed at a constant rate, or in intense short bursts after warming up, referred to as high intensity interval training (HIIT). Recommended guidelines for constant-level exercise suggest engaging in sessions of moderate intensity continuous training (MICT) for a total of 150 min/wk, usually spread over five sessions. MICT is any type of physical exercise that is undertaken at a constant rate without breaks, that raises your heart rate and makes you breathe faster, but still allows you to talk.

For HIIT the recommended guidelines are for three twenty-five-minute sessions, making a total of 75 min/wk.[21,142,143] A HIIT session typically comprises four intervals of four minutes at 85 to 95 per cent of maximum heart rate, normally after warming up, interspersed with three minutes of activity at 60 to 70 per cent of maximum heart rate. HIIT is more time-efficient than MICT, as calories are burnt at a faster rate.[144] HIIT may also be more enjoyable than MICT and a good option for people who are time-constrained or who can only manage short bursts of exercise at any given time.[145] It is recommended, however, to check with your doctor if you are not used to exercise, or have any underlying health conditions that restrict your ability to exercise, before you embark on a new workout regime.

Maxing out

The benefits of exercising plateau at approximately 150 min/wk for HIIT and 300 min/wk for MICT.[21,135] If excessive amounts of time are spent exercising or routines are strenuous, you need to ensure that you build in sufficient recovery periods along with the correct nutritional support for your workout schedule. Be careful not to stress and wear out your joints by overdoing it. Fitness instructors or health care professionals can offer invaluable support and guidance.

Weight training

Introducing weight training programme days alongside cardiovascular workout days can be beneficial in helping to achieve specific weight and health goals. It is worth noting that with cardiovascular exercise, calories are burnt *during* the workout period. The body stops burning calories soon after the exercise routine comes to an end. With weight training, however, as muscle mass increases you will continue to burn relatively more calories at rest, as long as the increase in muscle mass is maintained. It helps to remember that the largest muscles are in your legs and back. Training routines that focus on these larger muscle groups along with complex movements which involve several muscle groups, will lead to more calories being burnt. Most muscle gain occurs during the rest period following exercise, and not during the process of working out, which simply acts as the stimulus, so a recovery phase after strength training is important.

Working out with heavy weights can put a great strain on muscles and joints, so recovery periods of forty-eight hours are generally recommended for any muscle group you have exercised. *Do not be tempted to ignore this*, otherwise injury will force you to rest, and you may be inadvertently storing up problems for the future as your joints and back start to suffer from wear and tear. To improve strength, it is recommended using weights that you are comfortable with for at least two days a week.[143] Fuelling your workouts and post-exercise recovery period with nutritious foods can help maximise any gains.

Changing habits

In a busy life, changing routines can be helpful in providing the exercise you need. For example, consider walking upstairs rather than taking the escalator or lift, go for a walk in your lunch break after eating, get off the bus a little before your stop or walk to the local shop rather than drive. At home, domestic chores such as vacuum cleaning and gardening can also help you build up a healthy sweat.

Even low amounts of moderate exercise, such as fifteen minutes of walking per day, are associated with improved health and a longer life when compared to a sedentary lifestyle. Undertaking half the level of recommended exercise alone could give almost two years of extra life.[135] Also there is flexibility in how the recommended exercise levels are reached. For example, it is OK to perform activities in multiple short bouts of at least ten minutes, to get a person up to the 150 min/wk for MICT.

People who cannot manage the full recommended physical activity levels on account of health conditions need not worry. Walking, dancing, gardening, swimming and household chores are all recognised in the list of activities that count towards the weekly total for those over the age of sixty-five. Individuals with disabilities should try to be as physically active as their condition allows. If you are struggling with exercise, take medical advice before striving to achieve the recommended levels of physical activity.

Yoga and Tai Chi

Activities such as yoga and tai chi have demonstrable health benefits in achieving and maintaining personal well-being that should not be overlooked. They also provide the benefits of social interaction and cognitive stimulation of the brain which learning new routines bring. In addition, they can supply an ideal excuse to get out of the house and grab some *me time*.

Yoga is an age-old discipline, primarily designed to bring balance and health to the physical, mental and emotional dimensions of a person. It has become increasingly popular in the west. Yoga typically contains gentle stretching exercises and slow movements that are often coordinated with breathing, with the emphasis being placed on bringing full awareness to what is being done *now*. Regular practice can lead to increased flexibility, muscle strength and tone, along with improved athletic performance and vitality.[146] In addition, there is emerging evidence to support its use in treating anxiety, depression, sleep disorders, as well as obsessive-compulsive disorders.[147,148] It has been shown that after yoga practice, certain chemicals can increase in the body which boost mood and counteract depression. Yoga has been shown to improve mood and reduce anxiety more than other activities such as walking.[149] Specialised yoga designed for back problems can improve function and help reduce chronic back pain.[150] It should be noted, however, that although yoga has been associated with reducing high blood pressure and improving the health of the heart, it does not replace the need for cardiovascular exercise.[146,151]

Tai chi is the practice of slow and gentle movements combined with deep breathing and relaxation. It was originally developed as a martial art in thirteenth-century China. Today it is widely practised around the world as a health-promoting activity. In my local hospital, along with traditional medical treatments, it has been used for many years as a healing therapy to help lower blood pressure and heart rate after heart attacks, which is important in reducing the risk of further coronary events.[152–154]

Tai chi has also been associated with reducing stress, improving balance and mobility, as well as increasing muscle strength, particularly in the lower limbs. Many tai chi movements can be adapted to people with disabilities, including wheelchair users. Numerous positive outcomes are associated with tai chi, including improved bone health, cardiovascular fitness, increased physical function, prevention of falls – related to improved balance – and better quality of life as a result of reduced anxiety and depression, particularly when compared to sedentary adults.[152–154]

Exercise routines and techniques such as tai chi and yoga can help you reconnect to what is happening *now* in your life rather than needlessly reliving the past or worrying about what is yet to come. Mind-wandering has been shown to be directly linked with the degree of unhappiness you experience.[134] Your ability to stay *present* and focused on what is happening *now* is arguably the most important skill to have and nurture in life. It is only when you can befriend and settle into the *now* that you can actually start to switch off, recharge and enjoy your *me time* free of guilt, and the internal nagging critic that constantly harps on about what you still have to do. You can nurture the skill of remaining *present* by starting to reconnect to what is going on in *this moment* and utilising your powerful mind only when required for a practical task or purpose.

Living in the *now*

It is not uncommon to spend time rushing from one task to another and focusing on what needs to be done next, rather than what requires your undivided attention now. It is so easy to start drifting away from *this moment* and start thinking about the 'to-do' list. It takes practice and patience to learn the skill of settling into the *now*, but it is an essential tool to have in order to avoid mental and physical exhaustion, and eventually illness.

Learning to switch off the autopilot and to re-engage with activities and tasks in the *now* is life-changing. Rather than procrastinating about what is still to be done, lamenting about the past, or needlessly worrying about the future, see if you can stay focused on *this moment* instead as you go from one place to another.

How long can you use your senses to keep yourself in the *present* by watching and listening to something around you, rather than being lost in thought? For example, take something that many people take for granted, such as walking. Next time you are on some stairs or walking somewhere, see how far you can walk before your mind drifts off from the *now* to an unrelated thought. Research has shown that personal happiness correlates with the ability to stay *present* and focused on what is required *now*.[134] The seemingly superficial exercise below will not only give you an idea of your current ability to stay *present*, but can make you increasingly skilful in staying rooted in the *now*. Next time you plan to walk somewhere:

- breathe into and then out of the chest and begin walking
- focus on any sensations in your feet and any sounds they make as you walk
- see if you can feel any other sensations that are already in your body
- feel your breath as it enters and then leaves your chest
- as you walk, feel your movements and the contact with any clothes that you are wearing
- feel your weight shifting from one foot to the other
- use your senses to see, hear and smell anything that is around you
- try to walk with an air of openness and curiosity

- if your mind distracts you with an unrelated thought, take a breath and gently steer the mind back to what you are doing now

You can add a twist to this exercise. When you are alone, stop walking when an unrelated thought creeps into your mind and start walking again when it passes, just as if something physical were to cross your path that would require you to stop until it had moved on. This simple exercise can be expanded to any task you undertake, such as washing your hands, changing clothes or brushing your teeth. In this way you can start reconnecting with your immediate environment rather than being lost in thought. It provides the mind with an opportunity to rest and recharge.

Practising this technique will gradually enable you to walk longer distances without your mind-wandering as your ability to focus on the *now* improves. As you rush from one task to another it can be helpful to keep some conscious awareness in your body, maybe starting with your hands, feet or breathing as you practice this new skill, thus avoiding being trapped in the mind and compulsively following worry after worry.

Techniques that use sensory perceptions in a non-judgemental way to bring awareness back into the *present moment*, such as yoga, tai chi and mindful walking, are associated with a stronger immune system, the ability to have more fulfilling relationships, and higher levels of happiness. Although exercises such as the above may sound simple and superficial, research has shown that they can actually improve your brain and body structure.[155,156,157] Being able to focus on the *now* is what results in a happier and longer life.[10–13]

Summing up exercise

Exercise is undoubtedly good for you. It could reduce your risk of major illnesses such as heart disease, stroke, diabetes and cancer by up to 50 per cent, and the risk of premature death by up to 30 per cent. It can also improve mood, sleep, bone health, memory, and can be fun. Over the coming weeks why not try to keep yourself well hydrated, exercise, and maybe try some yoga or slow tai chi classes? Practice anchoring yourself in *this moment* as much possible and see how much better you feel for it.

I see many people who are desperate to add a few months, weeks, days, or even hours to the latter stages of their lives so they can be with their loved ones for a little longer. Do not wait until it is too late. Why not start looking after yourself now and encourage those close to you to do the same, so you can be with the people who are dear to you for as long as possible? Why not eat and exercise in a way that encourages good physical and mental health, quality of life and longevity for yourself and those people who are in your life? Individuals are sometimes so busy with the idea of 'making it', or get so disillusioned along life's path, that they give up the most important things: their health, well-being, self-development and happiness. You can be rich in many ways. A positive attitude towards exercise and food could well add quality years to your life. Your *me time* package to yourself should fundamentally include time for healthy eating, fluids and exercise.

Chapter 7

Me Time

Modern-day life can be frantic, hectic and time-guzzling. The day can easily be consumed and the years seem to fly rapidly by. There is always something or someone that requires your attention. Many people live in a society and culture where *me time* barely crosses the psyche. Even when time in the day does arise which could be utilised for respite, the internal critic does not ease up and internally rants that you can't stop. Even a five-minute break can soon come to feel like wasting time or being lazy in some way. The issue is that when people do things such as earn money, there is something tangible to measure. Cleaning the house, washing up, tidying shelves and gardening provide instant visible results. Unfortunately, however, when *me time* is claimed, you don't receive a tangible life cheque saying that you have earned another year of quality life.

The effect that continual stress and lack of downtime has on you may not be immediately obvious, but it can be measured, including the way in which it structurally changes your brain, weakens the immune system, and shortens the proteins attached to your DNA, resulting in premature ageing by up to a decade.[10–13] You may not realise how much damage a lack of *me time* along with constant worry and repeated low moods can have on your body, but over time they can rob you of vitality and longevity.[158,159] These adverse changes occur slowly, but you can start to see them gradually when you look in the mirror, at your waistline, or as health eventually deteriorates when something inevitably gives.

Me time is not just about exercising, healthy eating and staying hydrated, it is also about what *you* as an individual truly need to replenish, recuperate and self-develop. *Me time* can give you some much needed downtime so that you can reflect on and discover what you truly want out of life, rather than drifting from one day on to the next. There needs to be a balance between the pace and intensity of modern life and essential periods of respite.

The reasons why *me time* becomes difficult to come by and enjoy are complex. In the main, people are not conditioned for *me time*. Happiness tends to be projected on to some imaginary future point once certain academic, material, career or relationship goals are achieved, which fires up the compulsive thinking machinery.

It can cause excessive strain if people feel the constant weight of responsibility on their shoulders, or the nagging internal critic does not let up about the seemingly million-and-one tasks that need to be done. If you happen to find yourself with a few minutes to spare, an automatic reaction is often to reach for the mobile, laptop, TV remote, or vacuum cleaner. The mind is constantly bombarded by new information, past thoughts, or worry about the future.

Technology: friend or foe?

Advances in technology have produced a never-ending chain of must-have gadgets and status symbols. A new phone, computer, car, some form of new or upgraded can't-live-without smart device comes out, just as you have at last figured out how to operate the previous one. Fashion changes so rapidly that last year's trends are soon seen as 'so yesterday'. The powerful advertising industry never lets up.[160] A person has to be wirelessly connected by Bluetooth, Wi-Fi, 3G or 4G 24-7 in case they miss some amazing must-have deal or hot news. There is an intense and continuous bombardment of information and pressure to keep up, whether you are an adult or a child. Material completeness is constantly projected on to a future point as ads whetting the appetite are released before an item is actually made available for purchase, although there is always the lure of pre-order. You have to work harder each year as the cost of these items keeps going up. Everyone needs a certain amount of material possessions for comfort and to be able to function, but what was deemed perfectly fine one day rapidly seems to become obsolete the next.

Modern technology has made tremendous advances in communication, science, medicine, information access, and health care systems, but all this has come at a cost. The explosion in technology devices has resulted in 24-7 contactability, consuming ever increasing amounts of time that leave the mind on constant high alert. A person can be contacted at any time via text message, email, phone, pager, video calling and social media sites. People can even be tracked or hacked.

There is the increasing expectation of an instant response, as it is all about rapid turnover and meeting deadlines. The working day becomes longer at the expense of personal time for the self, family, friends and relationships. People are using traditional routes of sharing information less, such as writing letters or cards. Social networking allows for the instant sharing of pretty much anything, anywhere, and at any time, at the push of a button.

Modern-day technology has brought its own related health problems. For example, excessive use of texting or gaming can result in wrist pain, thumb tenderness, aching, numbness, hand spasm and difficulty with gripping. This is known as 'texting/gaming thumb' – the medical term for this is De Quervain syndrome. It is a type of repetitive strain injury that can be remedied with some rest, time out, and ice. However, problems are not limited to the hands. The WHO estimates that more than one billion people worldwide risk losing their hearing by having the volume turned up too high on devices. It is recommended that listening to music through headphones should be limited to one hour at no higher than eighty decibels, which is equivalent to the sounds of city traffic.[161]

Problems can also arise because of the sheer volume of information that the mind is subjected to, making it difficult to switch off. Information fatigue syndrome can occur as a result of material overload from text messages, emails, websites and twenty-four-hour multi-channel television programmes. The mind is exposed to an unrelenting stream of information from social media, news channels, family, friends and the workplace. It is estimated that the volume of this information traffic is now about 200 times greater than it was twenty years ago. Research suggests that it is the equivalent of trying to read 174 newspapers every day.[162] No wonder the mind can't switch off and people constantly feel tired! Information fatigue syndrome has been linked to anxiety, poor concentration, dithering, and a learnt obsessive-compulsive habit of checking for texts, emails and social media sites. This leads to a person becoming less able to block out irrelevant information, reduces productivity and the ability to learn.

Then there's the 'phantom phone vibration'. Being disturbed by a mobile phone seems to be an inescapable part of modern life, but up to 90 per cent of mobile phone users say they've experienced 'phantom phone vibration' where they think the phone has been activated by a message or call, but in fact it hasn't. This may be sign of overwork, tiredness, worry or insomnia.[163,164]

The internal biological clock may also be affected by overuse of technology, causing disturbed sleep patterns. As natural daylight falls in the evening the body becomes aware that it is time to sleep because the internal clock interprets yellow light as night-time, while understanding blue light as daytime. Modern LED screens and smartphone displays emit blue light mimicking daylight. This means that looking at devices which are not in night mode, can cause the body to think that it is still daytime, which may impair your ability to fall asleep.

It is a modern-day phenomenon that when people go out for a meal with friends they are often communicating with other people on their mobile phones rather than with the people whom they are actually with. The art of face-to-face conversation and communication are seemingly being eroded. When you are physically talking to someone next to you, there are relatively more hormones and chemicals released that help develop close social networks and have health benefits, than when you are simply texting.[165]

However, all these problems pale into insignificance compared to the stress caused by the battery running out, the recharge cable breaking, forgetting one of your ever-growing list of passwords, or, worse still, the device breaking or being lost. The price that is paid for this addiction to devices we carry everywhere with us is the precious life experiences we lose to them. A startling survey reported that 46 per cent of people said they would rather have a broken bone than a broken phone![166]

Take control of the time spent on devices, rather than letting them control you. *Me time* is not the same as 'phone time'. It can be helpful to have set times when you don't check devices, such as when eating meals, during conversations, at the gym, or after, say, 9 p.m. Placing your phone away from you, turning off all non-essential notifications, having a time limit in place, and leaving the phone in your bag or coat pocket when going for dinner or socialising, can help break any addiction. What about planning a technology holiday? Maybe for a day turn off all non-essential devices and have an IT detox so that your brain can relax and have a break. The world will not collapse if you do this.

Working smarter

The distinction between work and home life has become increasingly blurred as work can easily be accessed at home. There is an increasing expectation that work-related emails will be read and actioned outside of working hours. Answering work-related emails, texts and phone calls during family holidays has also become commonplace. Even going to the lavatory can be disturbed by the ringing or pinging of messages. This leaves the mind on constant high alert as the brain's fight-or-flight response system remains switched on, even at the end of the day when you require much-needed rest and sleep.

This constant pressure and resulting heightened state of vigilance has both a physical and a mental price tag attached to it.[167–169] It is therefore vital to develop the skill and ability to become *present* rather than worrying about what might happen, whether the phone may ring, or if work may send you another email. Too often people worry about decisions they have already made or may yet have to make, which distracts the mind and has an adverse impact on what they are doing *now*. This deprives them of the ability to get through the task they are undertaking *now* efficiently and then switch off even when there is some time to rest.[170]

As people work longer hours with fewer dedicated rest periods there is an inevitable impact on their cognitive performance and health.[171,172] There is a constant pressure to be more productive or work smarter, which essentially means to do more in the same, or less, time. Another efficiency drive is always just around the corner. Spare time gets slowly eroded, and whatever extra is given only leads to short lived grace before further demands are made or new targets presented. You start to notice that the same ideas or initiatives seem to come around in cycles.

It can be draining working all day and trying to keep up with the fast pace of change, modernisation, new protocols, new devices, and fresh targets or cost-cutting exercises. You can easily become exhausted and depleted by the time you arrive home, only to be confronted by a myriad of domestic demands as you don the chef's apron to conjure up a nutritious evening meal while holding back the temptation to use a fast food app.

Too often all your energy is directed at fulfilling the expectations of the people around you, with little time left for personal goals, dreams and aspirations. You can end up living a life dictated by other people, rather than one you really want, or set out to live. A dwindling amount of time is spent on activities you truly value, or things that are simply fun or interesting to you. Increasingly, your own well-being starts to become second place in life, and at times it feels like third, fourth, fifth place, or simply not featuring at all in the pecking order. It is like the analogy mentioned at the beginning of this book, where you are standing on a street corner on a blistering-hot day pouring out iced drinks for everyone who passes by, but in the evening when you are exhausted, there is not a drop left to replenish you. To go to the other extreme and withdraw from life without fulfilling any personal obligations and responsibilities is also not right or appropriate; this would cause unnecessary suffering for you and for the people in your life. The key is balance over the long term. It is usual to have periods of time in one's life that are frantic and manic, but problems will arise if there is no letting up of the pressure and if the demands become relentless. To carve out *me time* is not wrong; rather, it is meeting an essential and fundamental need for balance in life that all human beings have, and that includes you![173] Having healthy boundaries in place can not only protect you, but will help you to start claiming that much needed *me time* that we all need.

Everyone needs boundaries

It is very important to have healthy boundaries in life that are not compromised. You need a line in the sand based on your own beliefs, principles and choices. We all need this line for our protection and well-being. These boundaries define who we are and what we are not prepared to do or accept, in order to protect our privacy, dignity, morals, standards, health and *me time*.

Boundaries inform people of how you would like to be treated, spoken to, who you are and what you stand for. They help prevent you from being taken for granted or pushed to burnout. Setting healthy boundaries as you go through life that are not too rigid or too loose allows you to connect with your own emotions, needs and wants, as well as relate to the people in your life in a positive way. Boundaries enable people to feel safe, empowered, respected and be in the best place to help others in a fair and equitable manner.

Once you have established your boundaries, however, they are meaningless unless you enforce them. To do this you have to become comfortable with saying *no* when it is appropriate to do so, and that can be one of the hardest skills to learn.

Saying 'no'

People can continuously keep giving to the point where they become exhausted and ill. Some people can be so accommodating that they would never dream of saying no, thinking that it might be perceived as a form of weakness or vulnerability. There may be worries about letting people down or being harshly judged. For many people it seems as if keeping up appearances or maintaining that stiff upper lip is what it is all about, no matter what the personal cost or how it makes them feel on the inside.

If that sounds familiar, you are going to have to get used to saying *no* and sticking up for yourself. No one else is likely to do this for you. There is no doubt that saying no takes courage. There may be a perception that saying no is somehow uncaring, unkind or selfish. There may also be a fear of being disliked, criticised or risking a relationship, because saying yes is often easier and does not ruffle any feathers. However, yes may not be the right thing to say, particularly if you are already overburdened. To say no in order to protect yourself and those around you may be more appropriate at times. If taking on too much compromises the existing tasks that have to be undertaken, then this cannot be in anyone's best interest. Only the person who carries the workload knows how heavy it is, so you are the one who is best placed to judge when enough is enough, not the person doing the asking.

It is better to start with the small things when getting used to saying no. As your self-belief and confidence grows, you will gradually be able to take on the more challenging hurdles in life. The ability to say no is closely linked to a person's self-confidence, so changing what is going on the inside is the best way of changing your life on the outside. It is when self-confidence and self-esteem are low that people feel most wary of rocking the boat or potentially antagonising others. Bear in mind that the needs of others cannot always be rated higher than your own.

Coping with large amounts of work over the long term can lead to loss of productivity and motivation as tiredness, fatigue and exhaustion set in. Unless you speak up about the strain you are under – hopefully at an early stage – burnout can be waiting to greet you just around the corner. It is important to remember that it is the lack of rest and recovery that is the problem and not your ability to perform tasks.[160,172] Other people cannot be expected to read minds, so you need to speak up and tell them, in a non-confrontational way, how you feel as the opportunities present themselves.

Some individuals have an overt tendency to always agree to do things, so friends, family and employers may come to them first rather than someone else because they are less likely to encounter a no or be given a hard time on asking for more. If yes is always the only reply, the tasks that have to be completed spiral upwards, but the time in which to do them remains the same. Ironically, it is also often the case that the person who always says yes may be the one who receives the least amount of respect from others.

No one is immune. Many high functioning professionals cope for weeks, months and sometimes years with an ever-spiralling and unequal distribution of workload before it eventually causes both physical and mental suffering.[174–176] If a person is always submissive, demands will be made on top of everything else they have to do, including work, paying bills, maintaining a home, children and relationships, as well as keeping up with the latest trends and fashions. After all, one has to look glamorous while rushing around! There is only so much time in each day to achieve everything and working 'smarter' will only work to a certain point. Life can start to feel as though you are constantly chasing your tail.

Any chronic imbalance or excess pressure will bring with it a price to pay.[160] When things or tasks don't go as expected, criticism, guilt or regret can creep in because of self-blame and/or finger-pointing by others.[177] Most people can do such a good job at beating themselves up, metaphorically speaking, that they don't need anybody else to do it. Despite having a very convincing external persona that gives the illusion of coping, in the absence of balancing *me time*, internal suffering will set in, followed by visible cracks on the outside. Your material wealth, intelligence or who you are cannot protect you from these problems if you have not learnt how to say no.

How to say no

Saying no sounds so straightforward, and for some it rolls off the tongue effortlessly. For other people, however, this word can be incredibly difficult – particularly if they are a people-pleaser and having learnt this approach because it worked in their early years. It can be tiring, exhausting, and lead to irritation and frustration if all you ever do is say yes. Equally, you cannot go through life just saying no all the time. It is a question of balance. Saying yes to your responsibilities, but also yes to the things that replenish you, while trying to minimise the things that are draining can start to restore some order and balance. There is nothing wrong with delegating tasks and spreading the workload. A strong work ethic is important but you should not have to do everything.

Always ask yourself some of the following questions when demands are made: is there a win-win solution where everyone is better off, including *me*? Is there a compromise to be had that suits all parties? Am I being true to myself as well as to other people? Don't feel guilty about saying no to the children in your life either, particularly when reinforcing healthy boundaries. Try not to cave in if the guilt card is played. It is important for children to hear the word no from time to time so that they can develop a sense of balance and self-control rather than entitlement.

Guilt, fear and worry are often what drive individuals in the wrong direction in life and damages self-confidence. Beating yourself up and feeling negative towards yourself are acts of self-sabotage and should not be entertained. Although some people work better under pressure and with certain motivators such as deadlines providing the impetus to work hard, this way of operating is not for everyone. If you know yourself well, you will know what is right for you. No matter who you are, problems will always arise when the deadlines are unreasonable or unremitting and there is no balancing respite in which to recharge your batteries.

Also, consider these points: if you turn down a request you are not rejecting the person, only the offer, and saying no can create an opportunity for someone else to shine and show what he or she can do, so it can be an act of kindness. Don't compare your workload with what anyone else is doing or taking on, as everyone has different life situations, strengths and capabilities.

For those who find saying the word no difficult, certain tips may be helpful. For example, if you are not sure, say that you will think about what has been offered and get back to them. That provides you with some invaluable time in which to reflect on whether what has been asked for is really right for you. It affords an opportunity to discuss the pros and cons with the other people in your life whom you trust. Responses such as: 'I appreciate you asking me, but I am going to think about this and get back to you', or 'I am sorry but I can't help as things stand', might be the best response if you are already overburdened. Buying yourself some time, thinking the proposition through at your leisure, and weighing up the pros and cons, are good habits to follow. If you decide that what is on offer is not right for you, say no with confidence. State your reason for passing on the request and keep responses short but clear and consistent. Make it clear that all you are doing is safeguarding your existing obligations and ensuring that you'll be able to devote high-quality time to those tasks that you are already undertaking. Saying no at work and at home can not only be empowering, but frees up some time to pursue other interests.

It does not matter what anyone else is doing or taking on as people have different strengths, experience levels and life situations. If you have said yes to something already, there may not be space left to take on something that you know you would like to and will excel at. Another powerful technique to use when saying no is to breathe mindfully into and out of the chest; dropping your attention into the body and feeling the sensations that are already there. This can instantly reduce anxiety and help you produce a well-meaning and effortless *no*. Remember that you don't need anyone's permission to say *no*: it is your basic right to say this. Staying rooted in the *now* is a strong anchor that helps you stand your ground when it is reasonable to do so.[178]

Balancing the scales

Life has a way of coming back to the centre: the equilibrium point. Excessive work, stress, poor diet and a lack of exercise or sleep will at some point cause strain and suffering. Any chronic lack of self-care will be subject to the law of cause and effect, which will force a rebalancing of the way life is lived.[160] It is better to proactively restore balance in your life; otherwise life may compel you to do so. For example, chronic fatigue and burnout are associated with poor health. An illness can result in you having to take time out suddenly and unexpectedly. You have a choice; start restoring some balance now or wait for your physical and mental health to suffer and then be compelled to make changes in your life.

When any trauma such as an illness lands on the doorstep, it often forces a person to develop a new outlook on themselves and the world, because life as they knew it can no longer carry on. Any trauma, however, has a silver lining. For example, 90 per cent of individuals experience personal growth after a traumatic time or event.[179,180] A more resilient, optimistic and robust individual emerges. Often the worst thing that happens to a person turns out to be the best thing by acting as the catalyst for change, even though at the time the suffering may feel insurmountable and any positive talk seems like a flight of fancy. The trauma can act as a wake-up call, ushering in much-needed lifestyle changes. However, it is far better not to have to wait for any suffering to force your hand, or to keep putting off making positive practical changes to a tomorrow that never comes. Make positive life changes *now*, otherwise such changes tend to be forced on you, because life always restores the balance.[181] Some things will be harder to change than others but no summit in life is insurmountable for you, with the right action, concentration, effort, belief and intent. You can do this at any point in your life. Never doubt yourself.

In order to experience a healthy and happy life, there are two things you should consider doing. One is to try to increase the number of things that replenish, and the other is to reduce those that are draining.[182,183] Both are absolutely doable. Changes in life occur at varying speeds, but you can start to chip away at the things that are excessively draining. This creates space for new and replenishing activities to come into your life.

Practice being patient in the *now*. This will enable you to recognise and seize new opportunities and carry out practical and helpful changes to your life situation as opportunities present themselves, which they will do. Develop an idea of the direction that you would like your life to take, and what replenishes you. Sometimes people don't come to this knowledge until later in life, but it is never too early or too late to make discoveries about yourself or start to redress the balance in your life.

Over time you can start to shed what is unhelpful, unnecessary, unpleasant and draining. It is a gradual move towards taking on what you truly want in life, while reducing some of the burden along the way. Don't expect this rebalancing to happen overnight, or within the next week: it will take some time. There is often no quick fix. The practice of being patient often enables us to move forward and resolve situations as we encounter them in life, rather than rushing at things and thinking that they all have to be sorted out immediately. While being patient many of life's problems tend to resolve themselves. In days gone by, the practice of patience was considered to be one of the highest forms of action.

Boosting self-confidence

As soon as negativity or self-doubt tries to pollute your mind, remind yourself of all that you have already achieved, along with your strengths and core values. Don't entertain any negative thoughts or a critical head voice. No one can stop thoughts arising but remember that you have absolute control over which ones you choose to follow. Learning to watch your mind and not follow every thought that arises is a crucial skill to attain if you want to experience any internal peace. Imagine each thought you experience as a ripple in the water; following each thought is like falling into the water and being dragged along by every current that comes your way rather than standing safely on the solid ground of the river bank and allowing all the unhelpful and repetitive thoughts to flow on by. Observing your thoughts and following only the positive and practical ones is something that you *can* become very good at with practice.[178]

Another key skill is to start noticing what is actually around you now rather than watching what is playing out in your mind. If you spend your life blinkered by the past or worrying about the future you sacrifice the only moment in which you can actually make positive changes and find peace: *this one*. In other words, start making the *present moment* your constant companion. This shift in awareness comes from using your senses to become simultaneously more conscious of what is happening around and inside you at any given moment, rather than continuously mentally zoning out. Rooting your consciousness into the *now* boosts self-confidence and is the most important step that you can take in attracting new life circumstances and learning to say no. Quality *me time* is, in essence, befriending and being comfortable in the *now*. Like a heron standing on the side of a river bank waiting for an opportune moment to seize its prey, you will be able to seize your opportunities and make positive life changes while slowly minimising the things that drain you at home and at work. This only occurs when you become *present* enough to recognise the chances as they come on by.[184] New opportunities will arise, but unless you are anchored in the *now*, you may never notice them; hence the feeling that life never seems to change or gives you a break.[185]

As you become more *present*, life will start to helpfully unfold without you wasting energy on attempting to control or change things that are not possible to change, such as the past. Relaxing and focusing on just the one thing that can truly be done now enhances the quality of all that you undertake, and in itself is often enough to bring about welcome changes in your life.[186,187]

Living in the past will only lead to a low mood and worrying about the future only creates anxiety. Nobody would consciously choose these, either for themselves, or for their loved ones. Start making the *present moment* your constant companion and empty yourself of all negativity, resistance, anger and hate. If these emotions are not allowed to fester, this only leaves positivity, peace and happiness.[188] It is OK to feel upset at times as everyone has periods of low mood – we are human beings here to experience the full range of emotions that life brings – but it is best not to let negative emotions drive unhelpful and hurtful thought patterns, or allow you to become blinkered. Everyone makes mistakes. Reliving negative events only sacrifices the peace and calm that connecting fully with the *now* offers you, and which is rightfully yours to enjoy.

Chapter 8

Happiness Starts with You

Happiness starts with you, not with your relationships, job or bank balance, but with *you*! Research has revealed that it is not success that breeds happiness; it is happiness that forms the foundation on which success is built.[189–191] It is how you engage with life that decides on the level of happiness you experience; being happy in turn positively impacts on every aspect of your life.

As life progresses you can get stuck in a rut, overburdened with the amount of stuff that has to be done. It may start to feel as if you are sliding sideways rather than making any real progress. It may even start to feel as if each day is a carbon copy of the last, with nothing new or fresh breaking through. You may become disconnected with how things are now and start to daydream of a brighter and more exciting future. While you are mentally 'checked out', large parts of your actual life can start to pass by unnoticed. Research has linked mind-wandering in this way with the level of unhappiness a person experiences.[134] People who have an unhealthy preoccupation with events of the past experience low mood and depression. Worry and anxiety is coupled with obsessing about the future.[192] It is people who predominantly live in the *now* that enjoy the best health, prosperity, relationships and work-life balance.[193–197] Befriending *this moment* and connecting to what is going on *now* is the way to transform all your life situations.

The way in which people experience their own lives can be studied using brain-imaging techniques. It has been shown that people have two distinct ways of interacting with the world. One of these is often referred to as the 'default network'.

The default network

The default network operates in areas of the brain that become active when not much else is happening and preoccupying thoughts about the 'self' start to occur.[198] Instead of taking in and fully enjoying a moment, such as a breath-taking sunset, thoughts about what to cook for dinner and whether the meal will turn out OK or not start to creep in. This is your default network in action. It is the network involved in planning, daydreaming and worrying. This default network also becomes active when thinking about other people, and on holding together a 'narrative'. A narrative is a storyline about your life that is played out in your mind, like a movie is played on a screen at the cinema. The brain holds vast stores of information about your personal history which can be used to produce these mental movies. When the default network is active, thoughts about the past and future arise, not only about yourself, but also about any of the people who have ever been part of your life. You may start to play out in your mind what your parents, friends, colleagues, boss or partner once said, did or may yet do.

This default network, or 'narrative' circuitry, prevents any experience of *this moment* as the mind wanders repeatedly.[198] The more you mentally zone out of the *present moment*, the more active this system becomes, and the harder it is to switch off and enjoy what is happening *right now*. A compulsive addiction to needless mental time travel can develop so easily. An overly active default network can lead to you experiencing low moods, anxiety, depression, difficulty focusing, becoming blinkered, which result in loss of self-confidence.

The default network is active from most of an individual's waking moments and doesn't take much encouragement to operate. It is not good for your health to experience life only through this network. There is another way of experiencing the world, referred to as the 'direct network'. When the direct network is operating, several different brain regions become active. You stop worrying obsessively about the past or future, other people or the self. Rather, you start to consciously experience life as detected by your senses in *real time*, so that you enjoy that beautiful sunset as it unfolds and don't ruminate about whether dinner will turn out OK.[199,200] It is about using your senses of sight, hearing, smell, taste and touch to stay rooted in the only moment you ever have, *this one*.

These two circuits are inversely correlated. In the default mode you don't take in much real time information. For example, walking down the stairs when lost in thought is more likely to result in a fall or injury because you are not paying attention to what you are actually doing. Any resulting adverse incident is then often blamed on life or ongoing bad luck. However, focusing attention on what you are sensing *now*, rather than being lost in thought, reduces activation of the narrative circuitry and reduces the chance of that fall or trip. This also explains why, for example, if the narrative circuitry is going crazy worrying about an upcoming stressful event, taking a mindful breath can help switch it off as you reconnect to what is happening *now*. All your senses 'come alive' in *this moment*.

In order to interrupt this natural propensity to worry and attract threatening thoughts, step back and ask yourself, 'Is the situation really a threat to my personal survival?'; 'Is it worth the worry?'; 'Will this really matter to me in a few years?'; and 'What is truly wrong with *this moment*?'. It rarely is a threat; it is the mind that has gone into overdrive as your consciousness becomes absorbed into compulsively following thought after thought. The more promptly you can interrupt the brain's reaction to an imaginary threat, the quicker you can take action to solve the actual problem at hand and reduce the possibility of your thinking spiralling into a low mood and burning a permanent negative memory.[201]

The direct mode equates to experiencing life as it unfolds, enabling real time sensory information to be perceived, thus allowing you to get closer to the reality of anything that arises. In this way very few facts are missed, and consequently more accurate information is at the disposal of your mind when action needs to be taken. Noticing more real-time information makes you more flexible and proficient in how you respond to the world. It can break any hold that the past has and frees you from automated conditioned habits. You can then enjoy an increased ability to respond innovatively to an event or task, rather than just react in a predictable manner.

Switching gears

People who are mindful are aware of which of these two pathways is operating at any one time and can switch between them more easily, just like shifting gears in a car. On the other hand, those who are not conscious of these separate networks are much more likely to automatically take the default mode, which leads to compulsive thinking and worrying, along with reactive and predictable behaviour. People who score highly on mindfulness scales are more aware of their mind's processes, have more cognitive control, and a greater ability to shape their future by focusing on what they are doing *now* than people who score lower on mindfulness scales.[202]

Practising some straightforward mindful techniques can enable anybody to shift gears effortlessly. Being mindful is about learning to reconnect with what is happening *right now*. Any activity in life can be used as practice material, such as eating, walking, brushing your teeth or driving. See if you can stay increasingly *present* during these activities by noticing how your body feels and what you can see, hear, smell or feel around you. No matter how many times the mind drifts away from the *now*, repeatedly and non-judgmentally bringing it back to what is happening *here* and *now* will eventually tame it. Don't follow any inner critical voice that may declare that you can't do this, because you *can* with enough perseverance and patience. Consider one routine daily activity at a time, no matter how simple, and over the coming week start to bring full conscious awareness to that activity every time you do it. Then, every subsequent week, practice this technique with one additional activity. As the weeks go on you will become increasingly *present* during an increasing number of activities that were previously left to the autopilot. In this way, gradually more and more of life can be claimed back from the autopilot and experienced mindfully by reconnecting to what is being done *now*; staying *present* will inevitably become second nature to you. Practising while performing the mundane activities in life is what makes anyone increasingly skilful at being *present* in all aspects of their life.[178]

The key step to *me time* does not involve changing anything you do, just your *relationship* with it. For example, next time you are standing in a queue, rather than get irritated and run endless narratives about what you could be doing instead or berating how long you are having to wait, take a deep breath and have a break from compulsive, tiresome, blinkered and unproductive thinking. Use the time as an opportunity to notice what is going on around you. Be aware of any sensations in your body. Stay rooted to *this moment* by noticing how your feet feel as they make contact with the ground. Take some gentle, mindful breaths. Feel the breath as it enters your chest and feel your abdomen gently ballooning out at the same time. Maybe imagine breathing in fresh cleansing air and breathing out all that is troublesome to you. If the queue is not going anywhere fast, take as many gentle and mindful breaths as you like. Life will not come crashing down because you become *present* for a few moments and actually engaged with life rather than compulsively obsessed or worried about things that have happened in the past or might yet occur in the future.

Use every opportunity to observe and engage fully with what is around you. Listen to sounds as they arise without trying to analyse, judge, or wish that they were different in some way. Take a break from continuously judging everything; relax and take a minute to enjoy *this moment*, just as it is. A new idea or a solution to a problem is much more likely to arise in the absence of compulsive thinking. A person may even notice something that previously escaped their attention, such as an advert for the job they've been looking for. Being more *present* equates to being more aware of your actions and environment that will result in fewer errors, and in turn generate less fuel for regret or further worry narratives. It might even spell the end of misplacing keys, bags or phones!

Winning ways

When you use your talents and strengths, feel motivated, empowered and have the courage to seize your opportunities, you will have positive experiences and develop a sense of purpose in life. Success is not defined by a particular phase in life but is closely coupled with your happiness, which stems from the ability to stay *present*.[189] Your success and happiness are in your hands and not tied down to any particular life situation. The ability to stop engaging with the narratives in your mind, so they no longer distract you from what is actually happening around you *now*, is a skill that can be nurtured and developed by anyone.

Regularly look at, and adjust, the list of things that replenish rather than drain you. Start to readdress any fundamental imbalances, and in doing so free up some *me time* so that you can start to change for the better both what is within and without. Once you have made adjustments to your list, don't worry about whether the list is any good, if the things on it can be done, or run multiple scenarios of ifs and buts. Do the best you can, because that's all anyone can ever do. Stay rooted in the *now* so you can realise and seize your opportunities for positive growth and change as they arise.

Not being worthy

Guilt, fear or feelings of unworthiness can often enter people's thought patterns when they consider time for themselves. Do not allow such negative and unhelpful thoughts to settle and pollute your mind. The mind is like a magnet. A negative mind attracts negativity in life and in thought patterns. It is as if it looks for and feeds on melancholy. A positive mind, however, attracts positive thoughts and breaks the cycle of negative thoughts, emotions and feelings. So, stay positive about yourself and have faith in your innate abilities.

It is essential that you look after your body and mind, not only for your own well-being, but so that you can discharge your responsibilities to the best of your abilities. Taking five minutes for yourself so that the metaphorical 'reset' button can be activated is not a crime, but it can feel like you're committing one, particularly if it is not something that you have been used to doing. If the people in your life truly and unconditionally love and care for you they will support and help you with your *me time*. That arrangement should be reciprocal as they also need their own personal time and space. It is important to have a good support network and be surrounded by positive people who empower and help you through life's twists and turns.

There is a sweet spot in life, a balance where you can maintain good health and be well placed to take on all your responsibilities to the best of your capabilities. Always aim to find and maintain this state of balance, because in this life, no matter what is given, more will always be demanded of you, often beyond what is fair and equitable. It is not selfish to look after yourself, on the contrary, it is your basic and fundamental right. Do not let anyone take this fundamental right away from you. In a world lacking in truly mindful and self-aware people, you will be put upon, so you have to take charge of your own life, personal development, health and happiness.

Don't put the responsibility for your happiness in other people's hands; always keep it safe in your own.

Chapter 9

Relationships:
the Good, the Bad, and the Ugly

Just as happiness can be a positive influence, feeling lonely can have a major adverse impact on health.[203] In studies, people who report being very happy tend to have strong ties to friends, partners and family.[204,205] It has been shown that being in a happy relationship can be three times more rewarding than having your income doubled.[206] Sharing positive emotions, being able to talk openly, feeling understood, giving and receiving support, along with sharing life experiences, makes for happier people.[207] Healthy relationships support everyone's right to have *me time*.

A person can have many different types of relationships that often include friends, family, partner, associates, neighbours, colleagues and relative strangers such as the people who deliver the post, groceries, newspaper or milk. Enjoying at least one trusting and close relationship makes a person happier than any material possession.[206]

Then there is the most important relationship of all: the relationship you have with yourself. How you perceive your body, mind and self has profound ramifications for all that you experience in life.[208] The level of inner well-being you experience from self-development through *me time* is directly reflected in all your interactions.

Relationships tend to be a mixed bag. Some are uplifting, rewarding, warm and mutually beneficial; others may be hard work, and testing at times - providing plenty of fuel for building your character, resilience and resolve. The close relationships that a person has forms their core support network. The robustness and quality of this network can have a significant bearing on the level of personal growth experienced and the ease with which the inevitable hurdles in life are overcome.[209]

Life is cyclical, in that periods of hardship or loss are intertwined with periods of success and prosperity. A robust support network, which can include family, friends, associates, colleagues, neighbours and a close partner, is invaluable. To keep any relationship healthy, you need to do your fair share to keep it so. You cannot, however, form a relationship by yourself; there needs to be a healthy level of reciprocation. Relationships take effort, tolerance, understanding and time. Life's cycles and fluxes also occur in relationships as people and life situations change. Being rigid and unable to flow or adapt will cause relationship-related problems, including the one you have with yourself. A healthy relationship is a dynamic and constantly developing process as people's needs and level of personal development change over time. Being flexible, mindful and adaptable is the key.

You've probably already had varied relationship experiences, whether with your partner, family members, friends or work colleagues. Some may have been wholesome and positive, but others may have ended up turning sour. If there was a linear scale where one end was exhilarating and the other end bad or ugly, where you place any relationship can fluctuate over time and from day-to-day. You may wake up feeling quite positive, then someone says or does something and down the scale they drop to the 'bad' side. It is not unusual to have fluctuations in the way you feel about someone, and this often mirrors how you are feeling about yourself on the inside.

Opinions on what constitutes a good or a bad relationship vary widely. One person's idea of bliss can be another person's idea of a 'nightmare' relationship. However, some people don't know what a good, healthy and loving relationship is because they have never truly experienced or observed one. There is now, however, a substantial body of research that points to certain key ingredients that come together to bind two people in a strong, robust, long-lasting and fulfilling relationship: the 'good', as opposed to the 'bad' and the 'ugly' ones.

The good

Close relationships can provide some of the most beautiful experiences that life has to offer. Having robust relationships can support you at home, work and in carving out some essential *me time*. Unfortunately, there is simply no one magical formula that makes for a perfect relationship every time two people come together, as this is a complex and dynamic interaction. The robustness of a relationship will be tested over time by various life events, opportunities and challenges. People vary in their own level of self-development, resilience, effort and in their ideas of what a relationship should be like.

There are, however, some well-defined predictors emerging from studies of what makes for a happy and healthy relationship.[210] Certain interactions between two people strengthen, refresh, develop and maintain the closeness and warmth that every human being should rightfully experience and enjoy. Seven key ingredients can be commonly found at the heart of any recipe that makes for a wholesome relationship:

1. Compatibility: Choose wisely! Does your partner bring the best out in you, and you in them? If you expect and hold out for a compatible and satisfying relationship, you improve your chances of having one. Sometimes people are told that they are too fussy or they need to get on with finding someone because their biological clock is ticking away, but it is better to fish in a small pool, take your time and get it right, than rush and end up with someone who turns out to be completely incompatible.[211,212]

Everyone has the right to be unconditionally loved, respected, treated with compassion, and should have the choice in whom their partner should be. Settling down with someone should be more about when you are ready to do so with the right person for you, and not being forced into a relationship because of the expectations of others, or because you have reached a certain stage or age in life. Sharing and respecting each other's views on life, with the freedom to express yourself should be a given. After all, it is supposed to be a relationship and not a hostile takeover. Human beings are not possessions.

A good indicator of what life with a person might be like is the robustness of their existing relationships. How they treat other people, including their friends, family and colleagues, in addition to how they speak of them, is a good marker of how they may end up treating you or talking about you in the future. It will reflect on a potential partner's ability to nurture, develop and maintain a healthy relationship over the long run, rather than just superficially charm you during the courting or honeymoon period. It may also provide an invaluable insight into their inner state and the relationship they have with themselves.

High standards within a relationship are helpful, but only if there is a relatively low level of dysfunction and ego-centred behaviour.[213] High standards can be related to caring, supporting, independence, sharing core values and mutual respect. Giving and receiving is a two-way process. Before committing to a relationship, ask yourself some of these questions: 'How much do you complement each other emotionally, in interests, views, priorities and aspirations in life?'; 'Is there any chemistry?'; 'Do you make each other laugh?'. What can be better than being around someone who lets you be yourself and loves you for it?

2. Trust: Trust is arguably the most important predictor of a successful long-term relationship.[208,214] Is your partner your rock and 'go to' person? Can you trust your partner with anything? It is about being truly reliable and dependable rather than just saying that you will be so. The qualities of honesty and trustworthiness are essential. Be honest about who you are, how you feel, and your life situation. Everyone puts their best foot forward when they first meet someone; it is called making an effort. However, to try and deliberately mislead someone about who, what and where you are in life will eventually backfire. This will soon result in dysfunction and turmoil. A healthy functional relationship is built on a foundation of openness, probity, fairness and truthfulness. How can anyone fully commit to a relationship if they hold back about themselves in fear of being criticised or judged? If you are with the right person, there is no obstacle that cannot be overcome.

If you'd like to feel understood, then try to be more understanding and open first. If you want to feel love, then try to give more love. You have to treat people in the way you would like to be treated yourself, and then see how your life unfolds when you are fully engaged and trusting in a relationship, rather than hiding under a dark cloud of fear, worry or feelings of inadequacy. In any relationship there comes a point where you have to take a step of faith and trust if it is to progress to the next level. But this step of faith should not be blind; it needs to be based on what you have observed of that person's attitude to people, life, and him- or herself up to that point. Only then will you be able to move forward with a greater sense that it is the right person for you.[215]

A close trusting relationship has health benefits. For example, when cuddling someone, a powerful brain chemical called oxytocin floods your body with feelings of contentment and trust.[165] Trust is the foundation from which a strong bond can be built. Without trust it is hard for a relationship to grow and progress to more deep and meaningful levels.[208]

3. Communication: To keep any relationship healthy, it is important to be able to talk openly and communicate effectively. In a study that followed one hundred couples over a 13 year period, it was found that long-term couple happiness and stability occurred when couples engaged positively in attempts to resolve differences.[215] When you spend a significant amount of time with someone, sooner or later there will always be some degree of misunderstanding or miscommunication. It can sometimes be hard to air views without causing upset, but it is better to express the thoughts hovering in the mind openly and calmly than to keep things repeatedly bottled up, which can result in ill health and trouble further down the line. Suppression of emotion has long been suspected to have a role in heart attacks, cancer and early death.[216]

It may not go smoothly every time but practising open communication right from the beginning of any relationship will give you an idea of what long-term life with that person may be like. It is OK to have differences in views and opinions; people will have differing perspectives on life. You will have to agree to disagree sometimes and respect each other's viewpoint. There is nothing wrong with that; it is indicative of a healthy relationship. It is about being forthcoming with your views but also sensitive to the other person's feelings.

Right from the beginning, set regular time aside to discuss how each other's day or week has gone. Discuss any feelings, concerns, worries, or any recent highs and lows. In your relationship, make a habit of first discussing the positives and then the areas that may need attention. Always keep a focus on moving forward and resolving issues together in a constructive way, rather than just having a go at each other, fault finding, or practising one-upmanship.[217] It takes mutual respect, effort, understanding, maturity, empathy and compassion to communicate openly.

It is best not to play mind games or practice forms of passive aggression, such as the silent treatment, or to expect your partner to be a mind reader. If small things are left to fester without any communication, problems are guaranteed to grow, particularly when a release of all the built-up tension occurs in one uncontrolled outburst.

Try not to run internal monologues or dialogues while awaiting your turn to speak, thinking that what you have to say is more important than your partner, as they will sense whether they are truly being listened to and heard or not. It is always helpful to try and put yourself in someone else's shoes and see where they are coming from.

Body language is very important. For example, to frown, roll your eyes, or wave a finger is not good, as negative reactions can be unconsciously evoked.[218] In open communication, both partners should get an uninterrupted chance to fully express themselves. Closed communication occurs when only one person is speaking: a bit like a lecture from a teacher. Positive communication occurs when both parties involved feel that they have been heard.

How couples argue is a stronger indicator in predicting whether a relationship will or will not survive than what the argument was actually about.[217] The purpose of any discussion should be to achieve a mutually agreed and acceptable solution, not just an opportunity to yell about everything that has ever happened or take out your inner frustrations and insecurities on your nearest and dearest. If communication becomes difficult over the long term, marital support programmes may prove helpful.[219]

People communicate in different ways, and if you are with someone who does not understand that you need to be listened to, then that could be a lonely place to be! Communication is a very subjective between two people. Some people readily sweep things under the rug and are happy that way, but if grudges start to build up or issues are not addressed, then that rug will only hold so much before everything starts to spill out.

4. Positivity: A high level of positivity reduces conflict in any relationship. For example, the way people respond to each other's good news is very important. Excitement and pride rather than a sense of indifference, sarcasm, competition, envy or hidden jabs make for a stronger bond between people.

Being understood and validated, and with each partner feeling respected by, and equal to, the other, as well as feeling nurtured – irrespective of who is the main breadwinner – will bring couples closer together and strengthen their ties.[220] Staying positive and showing genuine care about achievements rather than just going through the motions is important, irrespective of the magnitude of the achievement.[221] Research has shown that in stable relationships there are at least five times more positive interactions than negative ones.[222,223] Both parties need to do their part. When this figure starts to drop below the 5:1 ratio, it is a good predictor that a relationship is heading for troubled waters, particularly if grudges are kept rather than practising acceptance and forgiveness. Good relationships are not a competition about who does what, or who is perceived to be more successful. Happy couples have the ability to learn and grow together through any interpersonal challenge. They complement and bring out the best in each other.

Find ways of developing and nurturing all your relationships. It is often the little things that really matter. For example, on interviewing couples, 62 per cent of adults say sharing the small things like household chores is very important for marital success, with intimacy rated by 70 per cent, and faithfulness rated by 93 per cent.[224] If a person cannot support their partner with the little things, how are they going to act when the more challenging troubles of life come to the fore? It is not just hard work and success that breed happiness, although they are both important, rather, it is happiness which breeds success and harmony in your relationships.[190]

5. Friendship: Being friends does more for couples than anything else and is a good predictor of whether or not a relationship is going to last.[225] Having your partner as a best friend makes for a happier, more romantic and satisfying relationship. What could be better than having your favourite person with you to share life's experiences? Closeness makes people feel safe and know that they can be open and honest, without worrying about being judged or feeling insecure. The more you share, know and unconditionally accept about each other, the stronger, more loving and loyal the bond becomes.

Does your partner bring out the best in you? Do you bring out the best in your partner? A healthy relationship should be like two supporting pillars standing firm and close together, but with some degree of healthy space in between. Everyone needs their *me time* for personal development as well as quality time together. In addition to the relationship with your partner, it is good to have your hobbies, close friends, and maintain family ties, otherwise it may become stifling and restrictive.[226]

Do you work with people who you genuinely get on with? Good social interactions at work along with job satisfaction is directly linked to relationship satisfaction and has a positive effect on home life.[227] If you have had a good day at work, the chances are you're going to bring some of that positivity back home. It is important to remember that although an occupation may be very rewarding, it is better to work as part of living, rather than just live to work. If you both have parts of your life that are separate, you both have new and fresh things to talk about and bring to the relationship. This will only work, however, if there is a solid element of trust between you both. Any insecurities may lead to envy, suspicion and feelings of neglect.

Put effort into building closer ties at work and at home. You never know when you are going to need your support network to help you through the sudden twists and turns in life. As well as your partner, good friends, family, associates, colleagues and neighbours can help you become more resilient, sturdy and better placed to cope with the ups and downs in life. In addition to increasing the quality of your life, a good support network can help you discover new possibilities and personal strengths.[228]

6. Variety: Variety is the spice of life and that includes in relationships. Trying new things and sharing new experiences keeps any relationship fresh and protected. Consider making a list together of existing favourite activities, and then make a list of new things that might be tried. Research has shown that couples who take part in more challenging and novel activities show larger increases in love and satisfaction scores, while couples performing mundane, repetitive tasks show no meaningful changes.[229]

Avoid getting into a rut and developing predictable habits. Make plans to do something fresh and different regularly. Set aside some dedicated quality time, once a week if possible. Consider a regular date night with your partner. Maybe even rekindle some of those relationship dynamics experienced during the courtship period when you were trying to win each other's affection. Why not do something spontaneous and make someone close to you feel even closer?

Sometimes a couple become too focused on careers, finances and raising children. They start to neglect themselves and their personal relationships. There is, of course, nothing wrong with focusing on children – they need you – but if both of you are not in a good place this will eventually be reflected in your family life as well as in your children. It is important to keep your relationship healthy and strong. One day children will grow up and start to live their own lives, and the 'empty nest syndrome' may be experienced. If, however, you have a healthy relationship with your partner, moving forward, you will find that once the children leave home, you will be able to use any extra time to strengthen your relationship further and explore new and enriching activities.

7. Happiness: If you are in a good place within yourself and experience well-being and happiness, you are *much* more likely to find success in love and life.[190] It is your attention, behaviour, attitude, compassion, receptiveness, interest and curiosity that are the genuine building blocks for a strong and healthy relationship. The more of these attributes you have, the stronger the relationship you can forge with another person.

Ultimately, the transformation of any relationship comes from within you, and expecting a partner to make changes that you have not made yourself, or are not prepared to make, is unrealistic, unfair, and is not going to lead to a thriving relationship. If you find inner peace and happiness, then this will be reflected in any relationship you experience. With your partner, you will either come together, if he or she reciprocates, or over time drift apart if one of you continues to self-develop and the other stands still. Either way, you will already have freed yourself from a certain amount of stress by realising you can only change yourself and that you can neither change nor control another person. If you find peace on the inside this will be a catalyst for change on the outside, allowing space and room for the people in your life to also change. Realising that peace and completeness come from a deep-rooted place within, sets you free. Don't let anyone drag you down, tell you cannot achieve this peace, or dim your light. Once you function at this higher frequency you will attract that which previously eluded you. Inner change is the catalyst for outer change.[178] Try it out for yourself and see what happens.

Don't place the onus for your happiness on to someone else. Take charge and realise that someone else cannot make you truly happy. Equally, don't make yourself responsible for someone else's happiness as this will only end in stress and frustration. You can be kind, thoughtful and loving, but ultimately you cannot be responsible for the happiness of others. That is down to them, just as your happiness is down to you. It is a fact that people who have a strong sense of inner well-being are the ones who have the best relationships. They are more likely, for example, to get married, stay together, and have harmony in their relationships.[208]

The bad, and the ugly

In the absence of some or all of the above key ingredients, a relationship is likely to experience some degree of dysfunction and become a source of stress, worry and upset. Periods of oscillation between good times and some form of negativity or falling out within a relationship are not uncommon. When conflict starts to become the norm, then there is a problem, and if some of the basic issues are not addressed, things can spiral into resentment and bitterness, which will generate suffering for all concerned.[230]

What once caused excitement, happiness, and was filled with promise can then so easily become tainted with disappointment, sadness and frustration as a person's imagined dreams about future bliss fail to materialise. Relationships are not just about the good times but also about supporting each other through the more difficult periods in life. A true test of a relationship is whether two people are able to back each other up when the going gets tough.

It may be helpful to remember that every human being has free will and that you can only truly make changes to yourself, and your partner can only truly make changes to him- or herself. You have to take responsibility for your own actions, but you cannot control, or be responsible for, another's. You can make suggestions, but ultimately the best way to bring about change, is to lead by example.

Manipulation can easily and insidiously enter the dynamics of any relationship, creating the illusion of control, but this approach only fuels further negativity as it eventually backfires.[231] If you have to manipulate someone, then clearly that person is not the right person for you, and you are not the right person for them. When confrontation occurs, remember that it takes more than one person to have a conflict; hence each individual has to take a share of the responsibility. Someone instigating conflict does not automatically afford the other person the moral high ground or excuse any ensuing reactive negative behaviour.

Non-acceptance is a relationship's biggest enemy. It generates negativity, bitterness and anger, which makes individuals become self-absorbed and only able to see one side of any disagreement. It prevents the acknowledgement of any good traits or positives that might balance things out. Negativity quickly breeds more negativity and is infectious. Try sitting next to someone who is angry; no words may be exchanged, but soon enough you will start to feel both uneasy and unsettled.

If personal criticism sets in, any aspect of an individual can be brought into question, such as mannerisms, character, behaviour, family, looks, ability to earn money, or performance of day-to-day tasks. People close to you will know your sensitive trigger points and how to 'push your buttons'. Often those doing the criticising or pushing are not in a good place themselves and project their inner turmoil on to others. It can be hard not to react when criticism gets personal. You can end up feeling upset, belittled and harshly treated.

Calming the waters

If someone is berating you, instead of getting upset or automatically reacting, take a gentle breath and try to understand what maybe going on inside that person to make them behave the way they are before you respond. Often some event unconnected to what is happening now has been bottling up inside slowly bubbling away, which eventually spills out in a negative way on to the people closest to them. He or she may have had a bad day at work. You yourself may have started the negative exchange; an unexpected bill may have landed on your doorstep or someone else may have criticised or treated you unfairly. Rather than take it out on the people in life closest to you, give yourself some time to calm down – maybe take five minutes and some mindful breaths. Accept what has happened and how it makes you feel, without judgement or over-analysing everything. Don't let negative feelings and emotions rise into the brain and pollute your mind.

Once your calm and empowered with some insight as to why you truly feel the way you do, try to discuss matters gently when the right time presents itself, in an effort to smooth things over and clear the air rather than letting things fester or boil over. *Never be afraid to say sorry.* It is not necessarily an admission of guilt or a show of weakness, but it can begin to heal many a wound. Don't listen to friends or family who tell you not to say sorry because 'you have done nothing wrong'; it is often the first important step on the road to opening up communication with someone, and for both parties to later have their say in a calmer and more positive environment. There are always two sides to any story. The sooner you start practising non-judgemental, two-way, open communication in your relationships, the better.

Remember that it is OK to feel upset. What has a beginning has an end, and that includes any cycle of upset. Accepting how you feel without over-analysing everything loosens the grip that any upset has over you. Practise being patient rather than adding to the turmoil; a bit of breathing space and time to reflect in a practical manner can calm the waters both inside and outside. Many of life's problems will resolve themselves as long as fuel is not added to a smouldering fire.

If anger, bitterness and dysfunctional behaviours are not nipped in the bud and start to infect your relationships, then what once gave you happiness may soon become a source of stress and suffering. This in turn generates more anger, resentment and bitterness, driving and magnifying any underlying tensions and problems. Relationships are a common, widely experienced and well-known source of life's joys, traumas and challenges. They provide fertile ground for a person to self-develop and grow.

There are many things that can influence how a relationship develops. Couples can grow together or grow apart. It may feel as if a partner has become a stranger rather than close friend particularly if there are different views on how to live life and conduct a relationship. Some people walk out of a relationship at the first sign of trouble; others may give it plenty of effort before calling time. People may also be dogged in their determination to save a relationship, staying beyond the point where it is healthy to do so.

The way a person behaves in a relationship is often related to the relationships they have experienced when growing up, along with social conditioning, stereotyping of gender roles, together with cultural, spiritual, and religious views.[232–234] All of these environmental elements, along with their genetic template, create something called a personality: we all have one.[235]

Personalities

A personality can be moulded by the nurturing and degree of family function or dysfunction that individuals have been exposed to in their early years. It can have a major bearing on their ability to nurture and maintain healthy relationships. Many terms describe a personality, such as: introverted, extroverted, compassionate, warm, fearless, hardworking, stubborn, lazy or easy-going.

Personalities are accepted as a natural part of being human. They can be fun, but when an individual's personality starts to interfere with his or her day-to-day functioning, rather than simply portraying certain traits, it may come to be described as a disorder. A personality disorder can lead to problems for that person and the people with whom he or she cohabits or interacts.[236]

Some personality disorders are more commonly known, such as Obsessive-Compulsive Personality Disorder (OCPD), but others such as narcissistic or borderline personality disorders (BPD) maybe more difficult to recognise. Certain aspects of these disorders are often portrayed in films such as *Girl Interrupted, The Boy Next Door, Gone Girl,* and *Fatal Attraction.* Often, however, the portrayal is one-sided as people with, for example, a borderline personality disorder, are often exceptionally enthusiastic, joyful and loving, but can be easily overwhelmed by negative emotions or the thought of rejection.[237] Hence the term emotional regulation disorder (ERD) is a more accurate description than borderline personality disorder.

The cause of personality disorders is not fully understood, but, as with many conditions, it is thought to be due to a combination of genetic and environmental factors. Traumatic events that occur during childhood may activate certain genes, which seriously impacts on a person's ability to regulate emotions.[235] Problems associated with a personality disorder may range from mild to severe and fluctuate over time. Problems are usually first encountered in adolescence, persisting into adulthood, but can present at any stage in life.[238]

Many people will have traits of certain personality types, but on average one in ten people will have a personality disorder.[236]

Responses and behaviour tend to be fixed, repetitive and rigid across situations. Typically, they are perceived to be appropriate by the individual suffering from a personality disorder, even when they markedly impact on his or her life and relationships. They may have difficulty regulating emotions despite an external appearance of resilience, and make frantic efforts to avoid real or imagined abandonment. They may also have unstable and intense interpersonal relationships, characterised by alternating between extremes of idealisation and devaluation. Experiencing an unstable self-image, impulsiveness, self-harm, feelings of emptiness and marked fluctuations in mood are also common place.[238]

When living with someone with emotional regulation disorder daily life can feel like an emotional rollercoaster. There may be frequent episodes of unprovoked explosive anger and paranoia. 'Walking on eggshells' may become the norm. One minute you may be considered as 'the best thing since sliced bread' and the next boring, lacking or inadequate in some way. A person with emotional regulation disorder finds it challenging to self-soothe and calm down. Many people may associate with some of these feelings and emotions from time to time, but when they start to impact on a person's day-to-day functioning, it is something he or she may need help and support with.

People with personality disorders may be highly intelligent, successful, compassionate, bubbly, warm, and fun to be around, but their emotional maturity has not yet caught up with their chronological age. Having an understanding of these disorders can shed light on some of the dynamics and interactions that are experienced in certain relationships.

Having compassion for others without the need to control or 'fix' them can be a very helpful perspective to have in life. If you know of someone who suffers from a personality disorder, their doctor should be able to help them, and there are many supporting organisations.[239] Regular exercise, adequate sleep, *me time*, a balanced diet, adequate hydration and stress management techniques may also be beneficial. It is, however, essential to realise that nothing in life is fixed for anyone, and that includes personalities.

Neuroplasticity

The brain and its pathways are not fixed as had once been thought. At any point in life they can be modified; this is known as neuroplasticity. The areas of the brain associated with conflict, emotional distress and worry can be made less active, and the areas associated with well-being, empathy and engagement with life as it unfolds can be enhanced.[155,156] Unnecessarily lamenting about the past, feeling empty, constantly wishing things were different from the way they are, or worrying about how things may turn out to be in the future, *can* be brought to an end. Anyone can change if they choose to do so!

There are various ways of undertaking these changes, including dialectical-behaviour therapy (DBT), cognitive behavioural therapy (CBT) and mindfulness-based cognitive therapy (MBCT), along with support from families, friends, associates and healthcare professionals.[240]

Anyone, regardless of who they are, can use these techniques to improve their coping mechanisms to deal with any emotional instability, and at the same time encourage more positive and life-enhancing thought patterns. These techniques help people to accept themselves as they are, without judgement or negativity, and they can help bring suffering associated with constantly wishing for things to be different than the way they are to an end. This empowers people to make changes in the way they choose to live their lives, from a solid foundation based on insight, trust and acceptance. Dialectical-behaviour therapy can help at least four out of five individuals with emotional regulation disorder and can also help their partners and family members. If someone close to you has this type of problem you can guide them to seek help, but only if they are accepting, have insight, and truly want to change.[241,242]

Nothing is set in stone

It is important to remember that, regardless of who you are, anyone can benefit from these techniques. Six to eight weeks of MBCT practice, for example, is enough to show growth in areas associated with well-being in the brain.[199,243] You can structurally change your brain. Anyone can become more resilient, and happier. Being mindful helps you experience a greater level of personal well-being, self-compassion and forgiveness. You become more productive and age less.[244] Mindful people are less likely to experience illness, worry and anxiety.[193–197] They are also more efficient, have a stronger immune system, and enjoy more fulfilling relationships. Mindful techniques can reduce anxiety, depression, overeating, insomnia and chronic pain, as well as boost the general quality of life.[193–197]

Being more mindful is about learning to use your senses to stay rooted in the *present* rather than needlessly mind travelling into the past or pre-living the future. Realising that you can't change the past and becoming more able to focus on what you are doing *now* is the best way to build a brighter future. The *now* is the only moment you ever have to fully live, enjoy and engage with your life and relationships when you are ready to do so. You can adopt these techniques and skilfully bring them into any aspect of your life, whether this might be driving, walking, talking to someone or washing up – just as we practised with that square of chocolate in the mindful eating exercise.

Trust, companionship, positivity, friendship, unconditional love and mutual acceptance of who you are and what you stand for should be a given in your close relationships. Many people grow together and experience a loving relationship where they are respected, share, enjoy and support each other through thick and thin. But what happens, and what do you do, if a relationship becomes one-sided, dysfunctional or you grow apart?

Chapter 10

Loving Me

There are many influences on a relationship. These often include finances, family, health, culture, religion, society, personalities, work commitments and environmental pressures. For example, the top five causes of tension in UK relationships were revealed in a study as being money, not understanding each other, differing sex drives, lack of work-life balance and different interests.[245,246]

It can be tough and lonely being single or socially isolated, so keeping your relationship with your partner healthy from the outset will pay dividends later on. It is about tolerance and compromise as well as enjoying the good times. For example, be open about finances; one person may be more risk-averse and want to put money away for 'a rainy day', while the other may be more focused on spending for today. A balance can be reached through trust, flexibility, open communication, understanding, and a compromise that both parties are comfortable with.

In a relationship, if one person feels he or she is repeatedly putting in more, not being appreciated, heard, respected, treated fairly or given his or her rightful share of *me time*, it can be a lonely place to be. If that happens, rather than one of mutual benefit, the relationship is more than likely to be a cause of heartache.

A broken heart

Often when people first meet a lot of effort and time is put into wooing one another. Sometimes, however, it is not long before that initial level of attention starts to wane. It may be that one person starts to make less effort or thinks that the other is asking for too much in some way. Some simply find that they cannot keep up that initial momentum and enthusiasm. People can also start to take their relationship for granted or begin to imagine greener pastures elsewhere.

What was fulfilling and exciting may then start to seem lacklustre, or as no longer living up to initial expectations, hopes, dreams or promises. People have varying degrees of commitment or effort that they are prepared to put into their relationships. As a result, some walk out at the first sign of trouble while others may cling on.

The end of any relationship can be difficult and challenging. A mixture of feelings can be felt, including anger, bitterness, betrayal, sadness, denial, rejection and loneliness, but also relief. While attempting to figure out how it all went wrong, poor sleep, difficulty in concentrating, comfort eating, weight changes, withdrawal, anxiety and a sense of vulnerability may be experienced. Blaming and finger-pointing may become a preoccupation. *Me time* tends to be brushed aside. A compulsive replaying of past events may start to occur as you imagine what could or should have been, instead of what was or is.

A 'broken heart' has been shown to impact adversely on health.[247] Friends, colleagues, associates and family members may also be affected. Even if people are deliberately unkind in love or life, you can minimise any negative exchanges and stress by not joining in. Unpleasantness often occurs when people vent their inner turmoil and pain.

Acceptance is freedom
Any separation process can be challenging, complex and upsetting. People vary greatly in their reactions. Emotions can run high and concerns over the future, finances, children and loss of home can propel the mind to think and ruminate compulsively. Bitterness, blame and acrimony can easily set in.[248] People may feel wounded and seek some form of reckoning and retribution, particularly if anger or hate is felt.

It is important to remember that negativity is a form of self-sabotage as it serves no purpose except to generate and perpetuate your suffering. Even if people do not join in with any mudslinging, they can unfairly find themselves on the receiving end of a host of unfair criticisms, accusations and abuse, as well as having to cope with any loss. How can a person protect and nurture themselves if such a turn of events is encountered?

The first step is to realise that these feelings are all perfectly natural and OK. When the bad or sad aspects of life emerge, it is human nature to experience denial, anger, an impulse to bargain, and eventually acceptance, when what has happened ceases to have a vice-like hold on an individual. However, to negatively ruminate is to relive life's traumas over and over again. In that way, events that occurred once are re-experienced many times, and that initial wound is only made deeper and more painful, which in turn takes longer to heal. To be able to accept what cannot be changed, but to have the ability to recognise and work on what *can* be changed is an important life skill to have.

At any point individuals can choose to accept their life situations for what they are, and their partners as the people they are. However, although acceptance means unconditionally accepting people for who they are, this does not extend to accepting any mindless behaviour, sacrificing one's personal happiness and *me time*, or placing oneself in harm's way. Acceptance refers more to what is happening *inside* you. There should be absolutely no reason to accept abusive, manipulative, or violent behaviour. Indeed, acceptance might mean recognising that a relationship is damaging or 'toxic', and the realisation that action needs to be taken to protect yourself and leave your partner.

When people behave in an aggressive manner it is a symptom of their inner turmoil and fear. It is a cry for help if you like, so retaliation is not the answer. A person who is internally in a good place does not behave like this. If someone is in a bad place and asking for help, it would seem insane to attack them, and sometimes people are in a bad place but don't know how to ask for help. However, it is important to remember that in any confrontation each individual is only responsible for his or her own actions and shouldn't project that responsibility on to the other person by saying things such as, 'You made me do it', or, 'If you didn't do *x, y or z*, this wouldn't have happened'. If someone in life tries to offer you something that you refuse to accept, it stays with them, and that includes any anger, bitterness and negativity.

Try not to get into any cycle of one-upmanship where the temperature continues to go up and up as you doggedly maintain your point of view, dragging up everything from the history books with no acceptance of anybody else's valid points. People who are insecure about who they truly are experience inner turmoil and fear. This fear manifests as anger and mindless behaviour. Complete acceptance of yourself and your life situation is what results in the complete and total ending of any self-generated suffering. It transcends the life event, prevents toxic thoughts polluting your mind, and brings your contribution to any negativity to an instantaneous end.

Focusing on the *now* enables you to connect to the completeness and peace within, rather than to any dysfunction and turmoil that exists outside. It is essential to carve out some *me time* to rest, recharge and reflect. If you and your partner are still together, *me time* also creates space for your partner to change and disengage from any animosity. You will then either resolve any issues and your relationship will excel and grow, or there will be an inevitable separation.[249] Either way, total acceptance of what is will instantly release you from any internal suffering, including any generated by your relationship.[250,251]

Resistance to what has arisen and cannot be changed is the bedrock of all suffering. Acceptance is the path to peace, freedom, a new life and a relationship that you truly deserve; a relationship that is not infected with dysfunction, but rather one that is built on mutual respect, harmony and unconditional love. Acceptance and forgiveness free you from the past. If thoughts of past traumas arise accept that they are simply fleeting memories being replayed, and gently bring your attention back to what is being done *now*, with the focus on moving forward and taking responsibility for your life, happiness and future. The *now* is the only place where you can build this better life, but you first have to fully engage with it to do so.

Taking a breath

Take a breath! You cannot lose your temper or practise one-upmanship and breathe mindfully at the same time, so get into the habit of burning away any negativity by gently opening up the chest on the in-breath and relaxing on the out-breath.[252] Initially it might be helpful, to count the breaths: one on the in-breath and two on the out-breath, up to ten, particularly if the inner critic has gone into overdrive. It also provides you with some space to respond mindfully rather than react unconsciously. Try it next time you are about to lose your cool. Notice how your breathing becomes shallower during a stressful situation and that you then reach a point where you hold your breath. At this point you often launch into some form of negative exchange.[252] Taking in a deep breath halts the descent into any negativity. You cannot get angry and breathe mindfully at the same time: try it – put it to the test. A little practice, patience and trust in yourself is all that is required to develop this skill.

If a relationship turns sour, you don't have to turn sour too. At any point you can stop your contribution to any animosity. Unconditional acceptance makes the decision easier as to whether to stay and work things out or leave. If you are in harm's way, then there is no debating it; this is unacceptable and you need to vote with your feet!

Next time someone is getting angry, imagine you are standing with a canister in each hand: one full of fuel and the other a fire extinguisher. Imagine that the upset is now a small fire. You can either choose to throw that can of fuel into the mix by joining in with the dysfunction and setting the flames higher, in which case both of you get singed and suffer, or instead you can offer the fire extinguisher. By not joining in and accepting that the other party is not in a good place and may be asking for help is a wise insight on which true change can be built.

My story

If you strip away the superficial outer layers, everyone tends to have similar wants, wishes, worries and insecurities. Fear of the loss of money, health, home, job, reputation, looks or the people in one's life can dominate thought patterns and keeps one stuck in a particular unhealthy life situation. It can stop you claiming the *me time* that you rightly deserve as worry or feelings of not being worthy take hold.

In most people's lives some things turn out well, or better than expected, but others may become tainted with sadness, unhappiness and regret. These accumulated life experiences, both good and bad, can become 'my story' which can start to replay obsessively over and over again in one's mind and dominate one's conversations. If you are not careful, the bad and sad of what has happened can perpetually start to cloud out anything fresh and positive that is happening *now*. Negativity can set in and become an all-consuming constant distraction to life as it unfolds. Continually reliving the story of 'me' will eventually impact on your health, career, personal and family life. Sometimes the worst place you can be is trapped in your own mind.

Bitterness relating to the past can feel like a ball and chain that constantly holds a person back and prevents them from moving on to the next chapter of their life. People can become so blinkered by what has happened to them that it becomes their identity. At any time, however, this fetter can be dropped. The past cannot be wiped away or altered. It can only be accepted, and the lessons it brought with it used to grow wiser and more resilient. It is often in failure and hardship that a person truly learns something about themselves and subsequently emerges as a stronger person. The past does not define who you are now. It may feel superficially cathartic to keep on reliving past traumas, but at a deeper level it only reopens old wounds and causes ill health.

When bad and sad events happen, it can help to use your support network to talk through things and to come to terms with, and eventually recover from what has happened. However, if you keep reliving and discussing the issue endlessly, people around you will begin to feel uncomfortable and unable to help, and for these reasons may start to withdraw.

Don't keep on sacrificing the only moment in which you can truly influence the rest of your life: *this moment*. Rather than be consumed by future worries or laments about the past, re-engage with life. Make the life happen that you actually want to live by focusing fully on what you are doing *now*. Let go of 'my story'. Why? Because you deserve better!

A new chapter

Inner acceptance of how things are sets you free.[251,253] It means that you no longer associate with dysfunction within, or without. At this higher level of functioning you are much more likely to be happy, successful and attract that which eluded you before.[189,190] Fresh, new, more positive and enduring relationships can be forged when you grow wiser as a result of your experiences.

Sometimes, when something comes to an end, it is life creating space and room for something new and fresh to enter. Fear of change or failure, letting down friends, family, children and a sense of being judged, are some of the things that tend to keep people trapped in unhealthy life situations. It is natural and OK to feel this way but accepting your good and bad thought patterns just as they are, rather than resisting or compulsively following them, breaks any hold they have over you. This approach is far superior for personal well-being than resisting that which has already happened and cannot be changed, or trying to suppress thoughts and emotions.[254,255] When you feel down accept that this is the way you feel right now, but acknowledge that feelings, moods and emotions are temporary and fleeting, and that there is no need to dwell on them or beat yourself up for having them in the first place. When it comes to the people in your life, feel what you feel with self-compassion, but don't take responsibility for, or take on, their emotions and issues. Just letting a mood or thought be without over analysing it breaks any hold it has over you. Things may be less than ideal for now, but life situations are not fixed. Welcome change will come when you make space for it to arise.

At the end of the day, if something has not lasted it was not meant to be. It can be more helpful to put your energy and focus into empowering yourself and into making positive choices going forward. Any negative life situations can be used for personal growth and to rebalance things at new levels of resilience, grit and inner strength which are patiently waiting to be accessed within you.[256] Start carving out some *me time* so that you can get to know yourself better and realise what you truly want out of life. Within you is an ocean of inner strength that will enable you to conquer any obstacle that may arise on your journey through life. As you progress along this journey, you will increasingly be unable to recognise the person that you previously were.

If something comes to an end, take some time out and try to learn how you ended up in that situation in the first place, so that the future does not become a reflection or repetition of past unwanted events. Give yourself space and time to recover. Don't negatively ruminate about what could or should have been and recognise that it is what it is. Remember that the past cannot be changed, no matter how much you might wish it could be. Self-criticism is not to be entertained in any shape or form.[257] Hindsight is beautiful, but you cannot enjoy and move on with your life if you constantly have one foot chained to the past.

Keep an eye on the brain's autopilot mode, which wants to replicate things, because what is familiar seems to be comfortable to it, even if it is destructive to a person's well-being. Life reflects not so much what has happened but how you respond, rather than, react to it.[258] Positivity, optimism, hope, belief and forgiveness are the building blocks for the brighter future that you rightly deserve.

True happiness in any relationship comes from the realisation that it is built on the one that you have with yourself. True completeness comes from within and on accepting yourself just as you are. This includes any perceived flaws or pet hates. In this way, unhelpful thoughts lose their negative and nagging hold over you. Befriending yourself just the way you are is the catalyst for change in your life, so take charge. Only when you have a balanced, stable inner state, are you able to form solid, long-lasting and stable relationships on the outside. Otherwise, any relationship will be a direct reflection of the inner turmoil within you, multiplied by that of the people in your life. Your internal happiness is the foundation for success in life and love, not the other way around.

To find a wholesome relationship, first find yourself.
After all, you are the most important relationship that you will ever have!

Recognise that you can do this at any stage of your life; so if you are already in a relationship, realise that the completeness comes from within yourself and not another person. Everyone is looking for happiness and unconditional love, but too often they are looking in the wrong place. To experience unconditional love, you must first learn to let it flow and emanate from *within you*. Only then can you give and receive it openly in your relationships. You cannot experience internal peace if there is an internal wall of resistance, bitterness, anger or hate. The prime and most important relationship is always the one you have with yourself. Once this is nurtured and developed, your happiness and positivity will attract the people and material things that previously eluded you. The inner growth that comes through self-development as a result of *me time* sets the background to the eventual transformation of all your existing relationships and attracts new circumstances in life. Often there is no quick fix, so make time for you and your own personal development and realise that change will gradually come.

It is your right to have choice, trust, open communication, positivity, friendships, and acceptance in your relationships. You deserve to have someone in your life that understands you, likes you for who you are, and brings out the best in you. It does not matter what has happened in the past. You can start to nurture yourself at any point through adequate *me time*, and then go on to experience the warmth, love and longevity that a wholesome relationship brings.

It is essential that you discover what makes you 'tick'. Discover what you truly want out of life and then go and realise your dreams and the life you want to live. Don't let anyone tell you that it is not your right to have or do this. Live in the *now* patiently, seizing opportunities as they arise. You are stronger and more resilient than people give you credit for. Robustness, resilience, compassion, empathy and the ability to have healthy relationships tend to be moulded through childhood experiences. How you interact with children and what they observe, along with your own childhood experiences, have a huge impact not only on the quality of their life, but also on your own.

Chapter 11

The Early Years

Interacting with children can give some of the most rewarding experiences that life has to offer. There are also plenty of challenges and character-building opportunities that provide the raw ingredients for self-growth. Children don't come with a detailed instruction manual. In fact, more information comes with the purchase of an electrical appliance such as a microwave compared with when a parent leaves the maternity unit or a child comes into the care of a guardian. There is no return policy or money back guarantee. Although a person's support network is frequently relied on for help and advice, it is often their childhood experiences and conditioning that tend to influence the manner in which they, in turn, raise their children.[259] Here you have to bear in mind that no one gets everything right one hundred per cent of the time; this would be an unreal expectation. Raising children is not an exact science!

The parenting style that you grew up with, coupled with the expectations that culture and society exert, can strongly colour the perception you have of yourself. It can affect your views about how you should live, conduct your relationships, and what *me time* means for you. This exposure may continue to influence you long after you have become an adult, as your mannerisms, life choices, personality and relationships mirror what you have experienced in your early years. You may find yourself replicating the way you were treated and spoken to as a child. These early experiences can have a major impact on any individual's health, happiness and vitality.[260,261]

Although there is no instruction manual or magical formula, there is a growing amount of research into the effectiveness of the different parenting styles and how they impact on a child. Knowing these different styles may help you understand yourself, your childhood, and your own children more clearly. It may also allow you to make informed choices on how you choose to interact with the children in your life, and to become aware of how those interactions may affect their current and future well-being.

Being Mum and Dad

It is not easy being a mum and/or dad! How to raise children is not taught at school or in antenatal classes. Some people have strong views on the subject which they are not afraid to express, albeit frequently devoid of any evidence base. Others may feel perplexed, overwhelmed or daunted by the task ahead. There are four main styles of parenting described: authoritative, permissive, uninvolved and authoritarian. On the whole, children demonstrate the most positive development when they experience parenting that is high in responsiveness, standards and is pragmatic: the 'authoritative' parenting style.[262]

1. Authoritative parents. This parenting style is characterised by reasonable demands, flexibility, and healthy boundaries. Although there are high expectations of children, they are given the resources and support that they require to succeed. Authoritative parents tend to be consistent and strict when they need to but show flexibility when it is appropriate to do so. For example, when errors are made, they will allow a child to explain what has happened, and if there are mitigating circumstances, adjust their response accordingly rather than react in an automated and rigid manner. They offer consistent discipline and reinforce any boundaries that have been set, but in a way that is fair and takes into account all the variables, including the child's intent and motives.

Parents who exhibit this style listen to their children and provide unconditional love and warmth but have fair discipline and clear limits in place when it comes to behaviour. It is an approach that emphasises sensitivity, reasoning and being emotionally responsive in addition to high standards. The children of authoritative parents are much more likely to turn out to be happy, positive, self-confident and resilient adults with the ability to adapt to the natural fluctuations in life situations. They tend to be academically successful, have good social skills, high emotional control and self-regulation. These children learn to strike a balance between freedom and responsibility.[263,264]

2. Permissive parents. These share some of the characteristics of authoritative parents in that they are emotionally supportive and responsive to their children's needs and wishes. They also discuss issues with their children. Permissive parents, however, tend not to assign their children many responsibilities; neither do they encourage adult-led standards of behaviour. Instead, children tend to be left to their own devices when it comes to regulating their behaviour.[265,266] Problems arise when boundaries are set but rarely enforced, so that a child does not understand or experience the consequences of his or her actions. Permissive parents tend to ignore or accept 'bad' behaviour, and bribe children to comply with their wishes, often to avoid confrontation. Adults who were not given direction or routine as a child have difficulty approaching the world with confidence. They typically lack a sense of responsibility and remain immature in their thinking. There tends to be freedom without healthy boundaries, resulting in children who are used to getting their own way. An overt sense of entitlement may easily set in.[264]

The expectations and behaviour of the outside world don't always match with their lives at home and so these children often become frustrated when the world does not permit them to have their own way. A lack of respect for authority and a resentment of rules often develop. Hurting people's feelings, selfishness or even aggression may become regular patterns of behaviour. Later in adult life they often suffer from low self-esteem and experience a lot of sadness.[264,267,268]

3. Uninvolved parents. These parents tend to have very few or no expectations about behaviour. They show little affection and may even intentionally avoid their children. They often fail to supervise a child and are usually emotionally distant and neglectful. They may not ask about school, homework, hobbies and activities, or spend much time with their children.

Uninvolved parents are often so preoccupied with their own needs and issues that they may not even realise they are not providing the emotional support their children need. Even if they become aware of this lack of engagement, they continue to prioritise their own needs above the child's. As the children of these parents grow into adults, they may experience difficulty forming healthy attachments to people, including with their own children. Low self-esteem can easily develop, along with difficulties at school, behavioural problems and unhappiness.[264,267,268]

4. Authoritarian parents. These are well known for saying, 'Because I said so!' when a child questions or raises an objection to something. There is no room for discussion, no choices to be made, no questions answered, and no opportunity to develop the skills of negotiating, or of exploring why something is the way it is. Typically, authoritarian parents have high expectations of their children, which is good, but they are much less responsive to their children's emotional needs. Failure to follow rules often results in harsh and automatic punishments. Children of these parents typically have poor communication and social skills, and often find it difficult to make decisions.

Many children who grow up in an authoritarian family feel that their own thoughts, emotions and opinions are unimportant and assume a submissive outlook in life. Others may become openly defiant and rebellious, becoming hostile, aggressive and untruthful to avoid punishment.[264,267,268]

Knowledge of these different parenting styles and their associated outcomes can be helpful in not only understanding your own life experiences, but also in allowing you to make an informed decision as to which style you may want to adopt in raising the children in your life. It is always good practice to be flexible and dynamic in any approach, because every child is unique. Children have different personalities, temperaments and levels of need. They often require varying amounts of time, guidance and nurturing as they progress through the different stages of growing up. These needs may also vary widely between siblings. Just because a certain way works for one child, it may not be best for another. It is not about giving all children the same amount of attention, but within reason, giving the attention that is required to a child at any particular time.

Sometimes one sibling may feel that another is being more loved and is getting more attention. This may manifest itself as 'poor' behaviour. Good parenting explores insecurities behind negative behaviour patterns and then provides reassurance. This can only come from open communication, setting aside time to talk, and gaining a child's trust.

The key to keeping the whole family happy, however, is always to start with yourself. Happy parents make happy children. You must do what works for you and your family, not just for the short term but with an eye on the long term. Parenting is about nurturing, in addition to meeting the physical needs of your children. It is about smoothing the transition into adulthood by means of gentle guidance and good communication. Parents may become so consumed with the many day-to-day roles they have to perform, such as being cook, cleaner, taxi service, sounding board and personal organiser, that they sometimes lose sight of the bigger picture. Ultimately, it is about equipping children with as many skills as possible for them to transition, thrive and be happy in the wider world when the time comes to fly the nest.

Copycat behaviour

It can be helpful to remember that children tend to copy behaviours, mannerisms and actions, more than what is said or preached to them. Children tend to observe how a situation has been resolved by their caregivers and may then replicate that behaviour either in their play or later as adults when they try to make their own way in the world.[269]

Children may be inappropriately exposed to what is happening in their environment, including to what is being portrayed in the media. They may also become embroiled in challenging life situations, such as separation, divorce or bear witness to domestic abuse. Children often mistakenly take on the responsibility for anything that seems to have gone 'wrong'. Young children look up to and are totally dependent on their adult caregivers. They imagine them to be perfect, so during challenging life situations they may conclude that the fault must lie with them.[270] This can have a long-lasting impact on their self-esteem and happiness.

We all learn mechanisms for responding to our environment – coping strategies – from the role models around us. What is learnt in childhood tends to be replicated in adulthood, even when that environment has radically changed. For example, a person may move to a different country and come to live in a completely different culture, but childhood learnt patterns of behaviour may continue to be replicated.[271]

Some people acquire robust techniques to stay grounded because of positive childhood experiences, so that when challenging life situations do arise they already have good coping mechanisms and are more self-confident whether resolving external or internal conflict. At the other end of the spectrum, however, there are individuals who have not been so lucky, and, through no fault of their own, have acquired little or no coping strategies. They struggle with the day-to-day aspects of life, particularly when managing emotions, and adverse life events only add to their problems.[262,272]

Most people fall somewhere between these two ends of the spectrum. As children they learn varying degrees of coping skills, resilience and grit, but have also been exposed to varying degrees of dysfunction.[272,273] This may sadly include emotional, verbal or physical abuse. They may also have had exacting and overbearing carers who have placed unrealistic expectations on them, making them either overreact to situations, or become submissive. This type of conditioned behaviour can further reduce confidence and self-esteem levels. A submissive adult may take on too much responsibility in an attempt to please everyone, but this approach is doomed to failure as no matter how hard a person tries, no one can be pleased all of the time.

People may mimic patterns of behaviour stored in their subconscious, either because they were previously modelled by their parents who themselves adopted a passive coping style, or as a consequence of over-critical, intrusive and controlling caregivers, they may have failed to learn more robust coping strategies for a variety of negative emotions, including anger, contempt, guilt, fear and nervousness.[274,275] There are also some children who end up taking on the role of young caregivers, looking after parents or siblings. They may miss out on childhood experiences, academic opportunities and the ability to self-develop, which can impact on their mental and physical health.[276] As they become adults a lack of effective coping mechanisms may become a catalyst for self-destructive behaviour.

Secure relationships

Although traumatic early life experiences can contribute to the initiation of self-destructive behaviour, the lack of secure attachments is what frequently perpetuates it.[277] Individuals who repeatedly self-harm are prone to react to life's stresses in a way that reflects their childhood trauma, neglect or abandonment.[277] Imagine how much internal turbulence an individual must be experiencing to cause him- or herself harm by, for example, self-cutting. Often the connection to current problems is not realised or acknowledged, but past traumas can resurface at any time, even much later in life, when a new event reopens an old wound. People who repeatedly relive the past end up experiencing cycles of negative thinking and end up making the wrong choices in life, which result in further regret, remorse and sadness. They may feel guilty and sense that they have repeatedly messed up their lives.

Having experienced negative life events individuals may come to think that somehow it is their fault, and this only compounds their misery.[278] It is, of course, not their fault. At any stage in life, secure attachments can help to make people feel safe and settled, whether that be with their parents, caregivers, teachers or a partner.

Growing up

The transition period from childhood into adulthood, adolescence, is faced with its own unique set of challenges and opportunities. It is a time when individuals increasingly try to stand on their own two feet as part of the journey to full independence and autonomy. It can be exciting but daunting as physical, cognitive, psychological, social and moral changes occur rapidly. The move to increasing independence and freedom also comes with new responsibilities and stressors. Attitudes and perspectives can fluctuate rapidly. Close family members may feel they are suddenly living with a relative stranger as the adolescent brain seems to be wired for aggression, pleasure-seeking, impulsivity, and risk-taking.[279] A new person is emerging!

Adolescents may attempt to do things which seem very much out of character to gain the approval and acceptance of their peers, much to the bewilderment of their caregivers. They tend to hide any perceived weaknesses and exaggerate their strengths as they feel a strong urge to fit in and be popular with their friends. They may feel an overwhelming pressure to conform, and materially keep up, with the latest fashions and trends. It can be confusing times as young adults try to find their identity and place in a world that is full of contradictions, confusion and conflict. No matter what the external persona or level of resilience portrayed, internally adolescents may well feel insecure, anxious, and fear rejection or criticism as well as suffer from periods of low self-esteem. These negative feelings and thoughts may lead to unprovoked verbal outbursts. Walking on eggshells may become commonplace as emerging adults can begin to challenge their caregivers' cultural and religious views and look for alternative sources of information which will almost certainly involve social media. Adolescent self-esteem can be easily knocked by any unconstructive criticism or by falling in with a dysfunctional friendship group.

The entitlement syndrome

Rather than learn how to accept and then come to terms with the way they feel without any self-criticism, escapism, along with instant gratification is often sought instead. In modern times instant gratification is readily available, for example, with posts on social networks that attract instant likes in an attempt to portray a perfect life and an air of coping.[280,281] Almost anything can be purchased by touching or speaking to a device, fuelling instant gratification. A product can be purchased and delivered direct to the doorstep without ever having to leave home or speak to anyone. There is little restriction on what can be bought. Permissive parents tend to give in continually to the demands of their children. Parents may also try to compensate for lack of quality time with their children by giving them material things instead. This can lead to a different problem: a sense of entitlement.[282]

If people receive pretty much anything they want, it fuels their sense of entitlement, and feelings of gratitude start falling by the wayside. An individual may be afflicted by the entitlement syndrome if they expect rewards for just being well behaved. As life becomes 'all about them', they struggle with disappointment and have the belief that everyone should run around after them. It can be difficult to restrain overprotective and over-pampering instincts, but that is exactly what is required to prevent the entitlement syndrome setting in.

People who suffer from entitlement syndrome often take things for granted and expect that if they wait long enough things will be done for them. If they hold out, someone will pick up their dishes, tidy their bedroom and do their laundry. If they ask enough times, someone will give in to their demands. If they act disappointed or sad, someone will give them what they want. People who suffer from entitlement syndrome place unrealistic demands on the people around them and learn to take more than they give. They find compromise difficult, crave admiration and adoration, and may punish others if they are let down. Dominating and manipulating others can become second nature.

To prevent an excessive and unhealthy sense of entitlement that may be carried into adulthood, a good place to start is to stop doing things that children and adolescents can and should do for themselves. It can be helpful to start with something straightforward, for example, if they are perfectly capable of washing and tidying up their dishes, they should, and need to learn, that it is their responsibility to do so. If they want the latest expensive must-have gadget, then consider meeting them halfway, or putting the money forward for the basic model and getting them to save up from their pocket money for the more expensive version. In essence, ask 'What do I want my child to learn in life?'. If it is the value of your hard-earned money, then don't just hand it over. There needs to be some effort made to receive extras, just as you have to put in hard work to earn the money in the first place. Children, particularly as they move into adolescence, can and should start to make some meaningful contributions to the household on a regular basis. Maybe washing the car or helping out around the garden will provide them with a little extra pocket money, otherwise they will soon realise that it stays empty.

Bank of Mum and Dad

If you go to the bank asking for a loan you are not just handed money; you have to make a reasoned application and plan any repayment terms. 'The bank of Mum and Dad' should operate in the same fashion. Children can use their allowance for 'treats', and as they get older take responsibility for school lunches, clothing and the cost of socialising. Having an allowance is an essential tool to help teach responsibility, budgeting, work ethic and how to save, rather than instant gratification and excessive entitlement. If children have their own bank account, this may remove the temptation for them to spend their money and provide them with an idea of how long it takes to save up for things. They are also likely to treat any items bought from their own savings with more care.

Everyone has to learn to strike a balance between spending within their means, saving, budgeting and giving. Children need opportunities to help them flourish and learn these valuable skills too; tough love is what is required. Guiding children should not be affected by whether you yourself felt loved or nurtured as a child, or whether you did or did not experience the best parenting style. Accept that you cannot change your past but that you can strike a balance between loving, nurturing and reinforcing healthy boundaries for the children in your life. Even if matters were less than ideal for you as a child or you ended up as a single parent, avoid trying to overcompensate with your children. At any point you can choose to adopt the parenting style and be the parent that you yourself wanted to experience.

The most important lesson is to learn to say *no*, and then stick to your guns. It can be incredibly hard for some people to do this because a yes is not associated with eye-rolling, fit throwing, pouting, tantrums or outbursts. Even if you are compared to other parents – 'so-and-so's child has this, why don't I?' – don't give in to the guilt trip. The short-term gain a yes brings will only cause problems in the long run. It is good for children to hear the occasional and appropriate no. You know that healthy boundaries are right, so hold your ground and breathe any internal discord away by gently following the breath in and out of your chest as you stand firm.

It may be helpful to remember that children are pretty resilient and resourceful when allowed to be. Parents may be reluctant to loosen the reins and let children develop the ability to be self-reliant but learning that rewards come through effort and hard work is an important lesson on life and in developing a good work ethic. To be considerate of how another person might be feeling, or what someone else might think about a given situation, helps children build robust relationships in the future. Children will surprise you with how much they can actually manage to do if they are allowed to do so.

Entitlement and instant gratification do not prepare a child for the corporate environment. In early adult life self-esteem can take a hit in the workplace where there is rarely instant gratification. Often in such an environment heavy demands may be placed on individuals, and the rewards can be slow to materialise, including promotions and pay rises. Also, there is no guarantee of actually receiving them. In fact, you can work your socks off and get put back or let go. In the 'real' world there is little or no pampering of anyone's sense of entitlement or innate 'reward centre', and young adults should be prepared for this.

The reward centre and social networking

The 'reward centre' is a collection of structures in the brain and nerve pathways where pleasure is registered and is responsible for reward-related behaviour.[283] There are many compounds that naturally occur in the body which when released activate the reward centre. If a reward trigger is repeatedly activated and left unchecked, this may result in the development of an unhealthy attachment. For example, instant 'likes' on social media sites can result in the release of feel-good chemicals in the body, such as dopamine, that stimulate the reward centre.[283] According to a study of Australian consumers by the San Francisco-based media company RadiumOne, social media usage is a 'dopamine gold mine'.[284] Addiction to dopamine 'hits' can develop easily and quickly.[285,286] Dopamine is also released during other activities, such as when a person receives a hug, enjoys food or during intimate moments. When people form friendships or have a wholesome relationship in life, however, they tend to get more of the additional calming benefits of in-house chemicals such as oxytocin and serotonin. The online dopamine effect can provide an immediate buzz, but overuse or over-reliance may lead to addictive behaviour and health problems.[287–289]

Any type of online rejection such as being blocked, or harsh treatment such as bullying, can have the opposite effect and cause stress hormones to be released. The UK charity Childline has recently reported an 87 per cent rise in contacts related to online bullying. The average time children spend online is currently three hours per day and increasing.

There is nothing intrinsically wrong with social networking. It is all about balance, just like anything else in life, and if used sensibly can have positive effects on people. However, if children cannot even get through a meal or short car journey without checking or watching their phone, or major distress occurs when their phone or other device is taken away, even temporarily, there is a real chance that they are suffering from an unhealthy attachment to their devices.

It has been reported that people who use a great deal of social media may have higher rates of depression and lowered subjective well-being, although the cause and effect can be difficult to disentangle.[290,291] However, if social media is used to strengthen and maintain social ties, such as with family members and close friends, it can have beneficial effects on mental health. Nevertheless, outside this use it may increase feelings of anxiety, loneliness, depression and poor sleep patterns.[292–294] It is crucial from an early age for children to learn about balance, self-control and having healthy time limits in place.

Social networking has caused a profound change in the way children and young adults communicate and interact with each other.[280,293] When sitting with friends, rather than learning to build relationships, they can be on their devices to other people. This can give out a message that, 'My phone is more important than you.' Parents or caregivers can lead by example by not doing this themselves; you often see parents of young children engrossed on their phones rather than interacting with their little ones, and this behaviour is being learnt at an early age by their children. Before you buy your children mobile phones, have an understanding in place for when and where they will be used, otherwise the phones may hamper their ability to have healthy social interactions and build the solid support networks which are important in experiencing personal growth when life's challenges inevitably present themselves.[293,295]

Cyberbullying is an increasing problem that can lower self-esteem and cause frustration, anger and depression. It can be helpful to educate children on how to protect and seek help immediately if any form of cyberbullying is encountered. This is the world that our children live in and it is not right to prevent them from being part of it, but it is crucial to equip them with good practices and coping mechanisms to protect their well-being.

Children and adults who have good self-control enjoy more academic success, better adjustment and less binge-eating and alcohol misuse. They have more interpersonal skills, form healthier relationships and handle emotions better. Research has not shown any negative effects of good self-control. On the other hand low self-control lays the roots for a broad range of personal and interpersonal problems.[296] Effort, concentration, the right attitude and self-control are crucial life skills to acquire, preferably in childhood, but they can be developed at any point in life.[297] It is never too late to change the style of parenting or yourself. Nothing is fixed as once was thought, and the cycle of perpetuated learnt behaviour patterns can be broken.

There is a balance to be had between nurturing and having healthy boundaries in place. Children will inevitably grow up to be adults and should be able to express their own individuality. They will test and explore their carers' limits and at times those of the world around them. A firm yet highly responsive parenting style is more likely to result in confident, happy and well-adjusted adults. In addition, there are many ways of overcoming unhelpful thought patterns and regulating emotions, such as the use of mindfulness-based cognitive therapy (MBCT) and cognitive behavioural therapy (CBT), with a mounting evidence base that might easily be taught to children and young adults. It is time for us to develop a practical *me time* educational programme to teach children from a young age how to build resilience, what makes a healthy relationship and lifestyle, and how to carve out some *me time* effectively so that they are best placed to navigate the twists and turns in life. Why not teach children how to be authoritative rather than permissive, uninvolved or authoritarian?

Chapter 12

Breaking the Cycle

People are adept at learning new skills and techniques, and once they are acquired, little or no conscious input or thought is needed to utilise them. It's a bit like learning to drive. Most people don't consciously think about driving anymore but can recall how hard it was when they were learning. You can drive from one point to another without any awareness of how you got there. As people go through life more and more daily activities are left to the autopilot, leaving the mind to wander, increasingly lost in thought. Eating habits, behaviours and environmental interactions, are often unconsciously repeated without any introspection. These learnt patterns of behaviour can be activated rapidly and mindlessly when the autopilot is left in charge. For example, if the autopilot senses a threat, it may trigger an over-the-top, reactive, angry exchange, rather than a measured or innovative response to a situation. Regret often follows such an outburst as conscious awareness kicks in after the event and an alternative approach or solution is realised only too late.

People tend to behave in ways that reflect their past experiences and conditioning. They automatically use the events of the past as benchmarks on which to base reactions to current or imagined future life events.[298] Society, culture, social media, peers, parents, teachers, friends and family can all help to mould a person's characteristics, personality and behaviour.

Blaming

We have all been exposed to some degree of unhelpful conditioning. It is only when we shake off our past and focus consciously on the *present* without judgement, negativity and with an acceptance of what is, that we can break away from repeating conditioned behaviour patterns and errors associated with the autopilot. When this occurs, fresh, new and original ways to resolve life's hurdles are realised.

There is no point in blaming anyone for your conditioning. Your parents had their conditioning, your grandparents theirs, and so on back through the generations.[297] It is all the same problem, forms of unconscious and conditioned automatic behaviour patterns that have been passed down through the generations. The important point to note is that this cycle can be broken at any point so that subsequent generations are not subjected to further unhelpful conditioning. *You* can break this cycle! It is never too late to change and to show people in your life, no matter how young or old, that there is another way; to respond and engage with life by being *mindful* and *present*, rather than reacting unconsciously and replicating the mistakes of the past. Leading by example is what changes behaviour in other people. The choice is simple: either choose a state of being by fully connecting to the *now*, which brings with it peace and happiness, or choose resistance, negativity and constant mind-wandering, which is associated with suffering and unhappiness.[299,134] The people in your life are likely to follow the choice you make for yourself.

If you start to become increasingly *present*, any planning is then practical, positive and constructive, and not driven by needless anxiety, negativity, rumination or worry.[300] It is when compulsive doom and gloom scenarios run in the mind, about what may or may not happen, that problems arise and health deteriorates. Worrying about how things may turn out is a form of self-sabotage. It adversely affects the quality of what you are doing *now*, thereby negatively impacting on your hopes, aspirations and dreams.

Wealth is not just limited to material possessions. A person can be rich in family, friends, health, career, happiness and *me time*. The foundation upon which to build this wealth is your ability to stay *present* rather than needlessly mind-wander. The degree of unhappiness children or adults experience in life is directly linked to how much their minds wander.[299,134] You can enjoy inner peace and completeness at any stage in life by befriending *this moment*, rather than lamenting about what has happened or worrying about what yet might be.

Rather than putting a massive strain on children with unreasonable expectations and a continuous projection of their happiness to a future point – for example, by implying that when certain grades or goals are achieved only then they will be happy – they can be taught to focus on the *process* of achieving these goals, thereby reducing their levels of anxiety. They will then be able to use their powerful and attentive minds to concentrate on what needs their undivided attention *right now*, in *this moment*, rather than be distracted by what may or may not transpire. The results then tend to take care of themselves.

To try the best we can, and in doing so become the best we can be, is what we all can learn to do. If we all put 100 per cent into the one thing we are doing *now*, it *will* immeasurably enhance the quality of everything we do, which in turn will positively impact on our future.

Having goals, aspirations, and dreams provides purpose to our lives, but it is focusing on the process that translates into better academic, personal and sporting success, rather than obsessively worrying about potential negative outcomes.[301–303] Children should be enabled to be the best that they can be, and not be expected to carry a burden of expectation that is unrealistic, or someone else's dreams and aspirations.[304]

A breath of fresh air

Mindful parenting has been shown to improve the relationship between parents and children, along with happiness levels in both. It involves being emotionally aware and non-judgementally accepting of individuals, but not necessarily accepting of their behaviour. It means listening with full attention and practising self-regulation, empathy and compassion.[305] Well conducted mindfulness interventions have been shown in studies and practice to address some of the issues young people face. Such interventions can reduce worries, anxieties, distress, reactivity, 'bad' behaviour and better exam results. Improved sleep, self-esteem, greater calmness, relaxation, self-regulation and awareness have also been reported.[306] It is estimated that more than a third of teenage girls in the UK suffer from significant anxiety and a quarter of fourteen-year-old girls suffer from depression. The solution to these problems can come by not only practising mindfulness, focused concentration, authoritative parenting, self-care, healthy eating, and regular exercise ourselves, but also by teaching every child these skills from an early age.[307]

Let's face it, life is never straightforward whether you're a child or an adult. Problems can arise, often out of the blue, some small, some big, some easy to deal with, some more challenging and complex. Given time, problems often resolve themselves. However, when action is required, the right intent, the right level of concentration and right degree of effort is what helps. If a complex problem arises, it can be helpful to break it down into smaller pieces and then focus on one bit at a time.

Anyone can learn to recharge by connecting with the internal stillness that comes with *presence* in the *now*, from where new, fresh and unconditioned ideas can originate. So, when a difficult problem arises, children can be taught how to connect with the stillness within themselves by learning techniques to stay rooted in the *now*. New ideas can then arise because the mind is no longer clogged with the grey clouds of worry and anxiety. If they cannot solve the problem they are facing they can always come to you for help and advice. Self-criticism, self-judgement or negative rumination is to be discouraged. If the problem doesn't require an immediate solution, it is OK to take time over it or ask for help. This is not a sign of weakness. If help is asked for remember that listening to someone also requires concentration.

Listening is a skill

Listening is an active process; it is not passive. It takes effort, attention and energy. True communication occurs when those having a conversation are considered equal. You have to remember that when you converse with a child the same principles apply, but you also have to take into account that they are still developing in the world and need relatively more guidance. A guardian or parent is not a best friend or peer, but a guide, mentor and tutor, particularly during the early years.

True communication occurs when people feel empowered and equal. If you have good communication skills they can be passed on. When people are talking to you, try focusing directly on what they are saying. Listen intently to their words, observe their body language, and try to understand the message they are trying to convey. It may be that a child or young person is trying to tell you something that he or she is worried about, or something upsetting that has happened to him or her. It may be that the child has finally mustered enough courage to tell you, in which case even if the timing is inconvenient, if you ignore them, or make the child feel unimportant, he or she may not try telling you again. It is important to realise when people want to tell you something that is difficult for them to open up about, and not brush them off, otherwise they may learn to keep adverse life events bottled up, which will only store up problems for the future. It helps to be mindful in all your interactions. The children of mindful carers are far more likely to feel unconditional love, and feel safe and secure.[306,299,134]

Unconditional love

The amount of self-respect, resilience, confidence and self-esteem people experience can directly reflect the amount of unconditional love they have received.[304] A person may have respect and love for their children, but it is how they *show* it that is important. A parent/carer is the first and prime role model. To show unconditional love, no matter what perceived 'good' or 'bad' things have been done, is the foundation on which self-esteem is built. It is important to remember that unconditional love refers to the actual child; their behaviour and actions, however, are a separate matter. All children need healthy boundaries in place which are consistently applied for their protection and safety. Loving people does not automatically equate to loving their behaviour.

When people start to become more aware of their own actions they realise that when children seem to be misbehaving, this is frequently a cry for attention, help and unconditional love from their caregivers. Empathy is when you truly put yourself in other people's shoes, to see where they are coming from before you respond. If children don't get a balanced amount of nurturing and guidance at home they may start to look in other places, or to people who may not be good role models. Children need varying amounts of attention at different times and some will be more resilient than others, so a parent will need to accommodate and manage individual needs rather than work on a 'one-size-fits-all' basis.

Children and young adults will tend to develop high resilience levels when they are protected by the positive actions of adults, by good nurturing and by balanced and proportionate attention. Ideally, both parents where possible should be responsible for their children's development. If this is not possible it has been shown that the most resilient children have a strong relationship with at least one adult, who may not necessarily be a parent. A strong bond can also help to deal with the potential harmful effects resulting from any family discord.

A person's psychological well-being, self-efficacy and the ability to engage socially play an important role in delivering high-quality parenting.[308] Hence *me time* is crucial to keep one's own resilience and batteries charged, in addition to creating some quality time when children can open up about how they feel. It will save a lot of future heartache if children can develop robust coping mechanisms and the ability to form strong social networks when they are young. Healthy boundaries can be re-enforced at any time, but this is best not done on account of anger, reaction or frustration. Practice keeping some awareness rooted in the *present moment*. If you drift away from the *now*, reconnect to your breathing or watching what is going on around you can bring you back into the *now*. The more mindful you are, the less dysfunction there will be in your family, and the more peace everyone will experience.[308]

Most people thrive and flourish when they are praised. Children know intuitively when they have done something worthy of praise. For example, if children have tidied something such as a cupboard or a bookshelf, explain that they have done a good job but also explain *why*. Consider saying, 'Well done, this will make it easier to find something when we next need it', rather than just saying 'Great job', in a rather off-hand, non-descriptive way. If the praise is specific it will carry more weight and value. However, over praising or giving praise that is not deserved may be counterproductive and devalue its worth.[309]

Family time

Being mindful is good for parents; it reduces negative emotions, including any pregnancy-related anxiety, stress and depression. Mindful carers report being happier with their parenting skills and their relationship with their children, who in turn go on to develop better social skills.[305,310] If mindful approaches were widely adopted, parenting practices would undergo a fundamental shift. The ability and willingness to be truly *present*, and to adopt a flexible approach to the constantly changing nature of a child's needs, will reflect upon the level of happiness that everyone experiences.

Quality time together can build strong family ties. Good quality family time can be enjoyed with parents, siblings and the extended family. This is not the run-of-the-mill day-to-day stuff, but real quality time where you do things together, which tighten the bonds that create a robust support network. Family time does not have to be lavish or expensive: it might be watching a film together, a family meal, going for a walk, playing a board game, a sporting activity, or a day out.

Encourage some regular time to sit down together such as meal times where devices are switched off. It is like anything in life, you get out what you put in. Society will hopefully start to put more emphasis into supporting, advising, informing, empowering and helping parents and children.

A stitch in time

Investment in terms of support, development and education in our children is crucial if we are to stem the ever-increasing health problems of modern day society. There are more problems now than ever before, despite advances in technology.[3] Children are often given the impression that happiness will be found at some point in the future, once they have achieved certain educational, family or social goals. There is nothing wrong with having aspirations, goals and wanting to achieve. They can give direction and purpose in life. However, to project happiness on to a future point is a self-defeating prophecy. It is happiness in the *now* and the ability to befriend *this moment* just the way it is, that breeds success in academia, sports and personal life. When people are happy and positive they are more engaged, creative, resilient and productive.[190] Happiness breeds success, not the other way around.[311,301–303]

Society places a heavy burden on young shoulders. Rather than teaching children how to be balanced and happy in the *now* – the only place anyone can be happy – they become conditioned, as their caregivers were, to project happiness on to a mystical future point that is never reached, because there never is or will be a moment that is not the *now*. Rather than befriending *this moment*, which is all that a person ever has, children are needlessly encouraged to time travel in their minds, away from the *now* to some point in the future, when they have done all their undergraduate examinations, degree, married, raised a family, established financial security and will then, it is suggested, have 'made it' and be happy. In this way there always appears to be a future more optimal point for happiness. This becomes a habitual way of thinking that causes unnecessary stress and pressure. That utopia point is never reached, so blaming the past and incessantly worrying about the future become the norm. People may end up worrying about life so much so, that they forget to live it. Needless time travel in the mind is the bedrock on which anxiety, worry, low mood, depression and self-doubt are built.[178]

The alternative approach is to teach people how to go about using their body's sensory perceptions to befriend and keep one foot in the *now*. If you want a brighter future, focus on the process of life *here* and *right now*, and learn to put one hundred per cent of your attention, when required, into any task at hand. In this way research has shown that results take care of themselves.[301–303]

If you want your children and yourself to do well
start to make this moment your constant companion in life.

You are then freed from the fetters of constant worry so that you can become the best you can be, rather than have your efforts constantly hampered by the weight of anxiety, overthinking and self-doubt.[312,313] Right- effort, action and concentration in the *now* will help you along the path to realising your dreams and living the life you truly want for yourself.

Parents have a golden opportunity to teach children how to achieve balance in their lives between studies, eating well, rest, work and play. Children can be taught how to perform to the best of their abilities, facilitated by adequate *me time*, so that they are fully charged, motivated and have every confidence in themselves to succeed. The art of practical planning can then replace needless anxiety and worry. This could not only add years to your children's life, but also add life to your children's years. Surely this is what all parents want?

'Quiet Time'

Mindfulness-based techniques in the classroom have been shown to reduce behavioural problems, worry, aggression, reactivity and anxiety, as well as improving academic success.[314] Students also benefit from improved well-being, sleep, self-esteem, greater calmness, self-regulation and self-awareness, along with an increased ability to pay attention.[306,315] Adults in educational environments may also benefit; for example, teachers trained in mindfulness have lower blood pressure, fewer negative emotions and symptoms of depression, along with a greater ability to feel compassion and empathy.[316]

Caregivers can explore a fundamental shift in their ability and willingness to truly be *present* in the face of the constantly growing and changing nature of the relationship they have with their children. To be free from egoistic, habitual and conditioned behaviour leads to a parenting style that builds an enduring relationship. Consciously selecting appropriate parenting responses that best deal with any current issues rather than mindlessly repeating the learnt reactions of old is what transforms any interaction into something positive.[305] Avoid the temptation to control a child and therefore to fail to take the child's wants, feelings and developmental needs into account. Instead, try to cultivate a relationship-orientated perspective. Remember that you were a child once and try to recall how people made you feel when all you wanted was to be accepted for who you were and how you were feeling. At the same time, however, bear in mind that the setting of healthy boundaries is something that should not be ignored.

When children are young it is important to give them some responsibilities, some chores that are easy to manage, along with constructive criticism and guidance about how to safeguard themselves, while aiming to keep instant gratification to a minimum. It will help to build their self-esteem and resilience in the long term. Show them how to regulate their own behaviour wherever possible, and this includes game consoles, TV and social media. It is all about balance and learning self-discipline with some adult guidance. Ultimately the best way to change your children's behaviour is to change yours.

An example of preventive action that has been successfully implemented has been seen at the Visitacion Valley Middle School in San Francisco. In 2007 a meditation programme called 'Quiet Time' was gradually introduced to try to meet some of the major challenges the school and its pupils were facing. Students were shown how to unwind and relax. Results started to be noticed just one month after the programme began. Among the five hundred students (aged between eleven and thirteen), it was reported that suspensions were reduced by 45 per cent and attendance rates increased to over 98 per cent, some of the highest in the city. Also, the rate of students graduating to a local highly academic higher-school rose to 20 per cent, whereas prior to the 'Quiet Time' initiative it was rare for even one student to be accepted. A survey from the state's education department found that the students at Visitacion Valley Middle School had become the happiest in the whole of San Francisco.

These impressive results have led to other schools in the US introducing the programme. Quiet time was developed to deal specifically with the underlying problem of stress. Students meditate for twenty minutes twice a day. Studies reported that the technique markedly reduced stress, anxiety and fatigue, and improved the ability to learn.

There is no reason why national policies and practices that support a child's healthy development could not be widely implemented.[317] In the UK over 400 secondary schools currently offer programmes such as the Dot B mindfulness meditation programme, which tends to take place once a week in personal, social and health economic (PSHE) education classes. Once a week, however, is unlikely to be enough, because it is only when these practices are brought into everyday interactions through regular practice that the desired impact is made. These existing programmes could easily be expanded into more comprehensive *me time* modules that also include other aspects of living such as: self-care, relationships, parenting, nutrition, health, exercise and using social media. A holistic educational programme should be an integral part of education systems.

Such a programme could play a huge part in helping our children and young people to navigate the complexities of life. The results of studies and research on how they can practically enjoy a healthy relationship, not only with themselves but also with their parents, siblings, friends and teachers, could easily be taught at minimal cost to governing bodies. Over seven years could potentially be added to children's lives with regular exercise and a balanced nutritional plan. Children can be taught techniques to cope with anxiety, low mood, and the stress of undertaking multiple exams while coming to terms with a changing body and mindset.[318] A holistic, all-encompassing approach is an essential investment to reduce the growing burden of physical and mental health problems which our healthcare services are increasingly struggling to deal with. It would not only add years to their life but also quality to their years.

Chapter 13

The Top Ten

When you are on holiday, you generally feel good about yourself as the pace of life slows, the 'rat race' is left behind, and you indulge in some much needed *me time*. You start to pay more attention to what is around you, the different buildings, food, drink, clothes, people and language. Time is taken to enjoy and appreciate what is being seen, felt, heard, smelt and tasted. It might be the case, however, that the people who actually live in the area you are visiting are taking all that you are enjoying for granted. Indeed, you yourself might live in an area where people come to visit which you, in turn, take for granted as you dash from one errand to another on autopilot. Wouldn't it be nice to bring some of that holiday feeling into everyday life? Do you really have to wait to go on holiday before you start to relax, try new things, and truly connect with what is around you?

As people go through life, there is a tendency for them to take on too much, but no matter how much they do, or how much they earn, it never seems to be enough. It often takes a complete change in mindset – which frequently happens as a result of some form of trauma or suffering – for them to start redressing how they engage with life. Suffering forces people to question what they are doing with their life and what they truly want out of it. A shift towards keeping things as simple as possible, focusing on personal happiness and health rather than material possessions, often occurs. People stop giving the trivial things more time than they deserve.

On changing your lifestyle, rather than going to task with, everything in life, it can be helpful to start to focus on what is happening inside you first. Maybe ask yourself: 'What is it that I really want in life?'; 'What makes me happy?'; 'Am I living life in the *now* or compulsively thinking?'; 'Am I constantly trying to be perfect at everything?'.

Are you constantly pointing the finger of blame or are you taking responsibility for your life? Regardless of who you are or what stage of life you are at, there are certain building blocks that form the foundation on which a happy and successful life is built. You can have happiness, peace, fulfilment and *me time* in this frantic world. Don't let anyone tell you that you can't or that you don't deserve to have this. Happiness is in your hands and not in the words of other people. It is time to stop making excuses. Don't let others hold you back from living the life you truly want and deserve. It is time to take charge!

As you try to climb up the corporate ladder and juggle everything else that life requires, the mind is constantly switched on, the body is not rested, and your inner self is neglected. Travelling away from the *present moment* becomes the norm, and the more you do it, the unhappier you become. Human beings tend to develop a habit of worrying and constantly feeling the need to be 'doing', with no balancing respite that comes with just 'being' and enjoying life as it unfolds moment by moment. It is as if the being part of human being has been forgotten.

Living in the past tends to drag up unpleasant memories without any balancing recall of positive events. Obsessing about what may or may not happen in the future brings not only worry, anxiety and uncertainty, but also the false promise of that elusive happiness that will come once you have 'made it'. Negativity towards *this moment*, and an inability to accept life as it actually is, including yourself, can easily set in. It seems as though there is always a gap between the way things are and the way you would like them to be. This imagined gap is the fundamental cause of suffering. If resistance to the way things are locks you into suffering, then acceptance is the key that frees you and unlocks your happiness. Acceptance is the first of the ten fundamental building blocks on which the foundation for your happiness and the life you actually want to live is built on.

1. Acceptance. Unconditional acceptance frees you from suffering, transcends all life situations, and sets you free. Rather than constantly berating what has happened or judging the way things are, accept that everyone is at different stages of their self-development. Let go of all that is negative and unhelpful. Leave behind the need to constantly judge, control or label because everyone has had different opportunities, challenges and life experiences. Realise that everyone is striving for the same things; acceptance of who they are, to feel safe, be free from suffering, and to experience unconditional love and peace.

Accepting your friends, family, associates, colleagues and social support networks just as they are instantaneously frees you from any relationship generated turmoil. It is only when there is a wish for things to be different than the way they are that suffering rears its ugly head. Your life situation may be far from ideal. Things may not have panned out as you previously imagined they would, however, acceptance does not mean that you cannot shake things up and bring about some welcome change to your current life situation.

Acceptance is more about what is happening within you, rather than what is happening outside of you. Free yourself of all that weighs you down and burdens you within, such as anger, hate, bitterness, frustration and resentment. Instead drive your energy into making positive and practical changes. Stay positive in your view of yourself and see how your life changes at this higher frequency.

If you want to see change on the outside, first change the relationship you have with yourself by accepting and coming to terms with what is within. Never criticise yourself in any way, shape or form. Don't give in to, or follow, any negative internal chatter. Instead develop positive affirmations such as: 'I am the architect of my life'; 'I will succeed'; 'I am loved'; 'I am worthy'; and 'Life has a perfect plan for me'. Stay focused on *this moment*, do the best you can, accept the lessons of the past, but never look back in bitterness. Inner acceptance and change is the way to effect external change, not the other way around. Non-acceptance just keeps reopening old wounds and blunts your innate ability to heal.

If something unexpected arises, learn to accept it as soon as you can, knowing that what has happened cannot be changed, because you cannot travel into the past and change the course of history. Once you have accepted the unexpected, you can put your energy and innate abilities into bringing about positive changes rather than wasting your precious resources on berating the fact that something happened in the first place.

It can be helpful to take a break and spend some time outside. Nature is a great teacher. It exists solely in the *now*. People who regularly enjoy watching and being part of nature feel their lives are more worthwhile and are happier.[319] Everything happens when it is time for it to happen. You realise that everything occurs in cycles. There is no lamenting the past or anxieties about the future. Nature does not take on too much. What is needed is acquired and the rest of the time is spent in just living life as it unfolds moment by moment. Spending time in nature can help you connect with *this moment*, the only moment you ever have.

Try not to accumulate any more traumas or difficulties as you go through life. Keep your life as simple as possible. Try not to over complicate things or repeatedly overstretch yourself. Life has a way of rebalancing and will force change on you if you keep yourself exposed to long-term strain. To accept and fully engage with life as it unfolds is like effortlessly floating along a stream of water rather than constantly fighting the current. It is healthy to have dreams, aspirations, hopes and goals, and by focusing on what can be changed, helps you realise them.

Accept that it is normal to feel periods of low mood or anxiety, particularly when unexpected and adverse change comes your way. Accept that everyone makes mistakes. People grow more resilient and wiser by learning from their errors. It is often said that your best teacher is your last mistake. If you want to make positive changes in your life then learn from the past, but always keep one foot in the *now* and step forward with the other. The *now* is the only place where you can take charge of your life and affect positive changes. Suffering is always the result of some form of resistance to what has happened or worry over the way things are or may turn out to be. Unconditional acceptance of all that is, including yourself, frees you from all the fetters of suffering.

2. Friends for life. Good relationships with close family members, friends, associates, colleagues, teammates and your partner are important. Giving and receiving help and support from those who care about you builds resilience and helps you to stay grounded. If you want to experience personal growth it is important to have good, solid, wholesome, mutually beneficial and respectful relationships. Strong relationships are linked with a 50 per cent increase in longevity.[320] Some people find that being active in social groups and organisations may also provide social support.

Ask yourself: 'Is my life full of "radiators" or "drains"?'. 'Radiators' are people who on the whole exhibit warmth, kindness, compassion, happiness and enthusiasm. Their glass is always half full. They smile when you walk into the room, are genuinely interested in you, and make you feel good about yourself. 'Radiators' bring out the very best in you. They may occasionally have their own issues when they also need some support, but in the main life is to be positively engaged with and experienced.

When truly awful things happen, it is hard to feel like a 'radiator' and you should not be expected to feel so. Some *me time* to recover and recuperate, supported by your social network, can be invaluable. 'Radiators' inherently tend to live life as it unfolds rather than lamenting about a long-gone past or being buried under layers of worry about what might happen, so tend to bounce back quickly. They realise that helping others also benefits the helper. They always look for the win-win in every situation so that everyone is happy.

'Drains', on the other hand, can zap your energy and generally take more than they give. Their glass is usually half empty. They tend to be focused on themselves and seem oblivious to the feelings, views or opinions of others. After a period of time with them you may feel drained, tired, exhausted or downbeat. The friendship may have been different to start with but may have changed over time. Sometimes the routine of seeing them is the only thing that keeps the friendship going.

Accept that you cannot click with everyone, but that you have a natural affinity with others and be OK with this. It is not a personal failing but part and parcel of life. It can be a hard decision to let a friendship go, but the chances are that if it is not good for you, it is not doing the other person any good either.

By letting go of resistance and surrendering to the *now*, anyone can become a 'radiator'. Having a core support network that contains 'radiators' can help lift you when the low tides of life seem to drag you along with them. As you go through life, build bridges with, and develop, a core network of close 'radiators'. The best way to do this is to dump negativity and become more positive, upbeat, and warm yourself first. You will then become what you want to be and attract what you want most in life.

A good role model and mentor that 'gets you' and helps you can also be invaluable, whether a teacher, friend, associate or family member. Although ultimately it is belief in yourself that empowers you, to have a good core support network makes life so much easier. Life is a long way to walk unaided, unguided or alone. Keep those who are close to you closer by mutually respecting, helping, giving them quality time, actively listening to them and valuing them.

3. Belief in yourself. Say no to the inner critic! Take stock of all the things you have already accomplished and are going to achieve. Realise that you are unique and that there has never been, or will be, anyone like you. Within you exists all that you need to overcome whatever obstacles life puts in your way. Having belief in yourself is half the battle already won.

At times, it can be hard to believe in yourself, especially when bad, sad or unfair things happen. Negative feelings and thought patterns may also set in, such as feeling that you have nothing to offer or that you are unworthy. People often don't need the outside world to beat them up as they do such a good job of it themselves. Hindsight is a beautiful thing, but exactly that, so if something happened that you come to regret, learn the lesson and leave it where it belongs, in the vault of the past. Don't needlessly time travel to relive and reopen old wounds.

We all wish that life could be a breeze and that no one ever had to face any upset, but we cannot change the fact that highly challenging events occur. These times, however, don't last forever, and experiencing, learning and coming out the other side as a more resilient, stronger and robust individual is what it is all about. On the whole life's challenges are fleeting and temporary, but you are not. So, stand your ground when any ill wind arises, knowing that it will pass and that you will emerge all the stronger for it. Never be afraid to face and take on your fears. As you begin to surmount the challenges you encounter in life, you will begin to feel more positive in your innate ability to succeed. You'll come to understand the fundamental cycles of ups and downs upon which life is based. If there were no challenges, where would the impetus to grow, develop and better yourself come from?

Have trust in yourself, as there is no obstacle that you cannot overcome with patience and perseverance. Be realistic in your goals and don't listen to the inner critic or any unconstructive negative people who try to hold you back. People who experience well-being and have the greatest sense of purpose in their lives live significantly longer.[321] To live the life you truly want, you must first fully believe in yourself and your innate abilities. There will be setbacks, but you *can* overcome them all with belief in yourself.

4. Taking care of you. Realise that you can't be everything for everyone. Accept that fact and be OK with it. Focus some of your time and energy on the things that replenish you. Taking care of your responsibilities and taking care of yourself are not mutually exclusive. Get enough sleep: don't burn the midnight oil unnecessarily. Start doing more of what makes you happy such as reading, listening to music, engaging in hobbies, going for walks, or singing. Fitting in some exercise can be easier than you think. For example, consider walking upstairs rather than taking the lift, get off the bus a few stops before you need to and walk the rest of the way, or spend part of your lunch hour going for a walk.

You may be extremely proud of how much you do for your loved ones, but this should not be at the expense of your health and well-being. A lack of balancing respite will eventually lead to tiredness, exhaustion and burnout. In the process of putting so much into caring for others, don't forget about your own needs. It is your basic right to exercise, eat well and have *me time*. It is OK to say no, delegate, or ask for help; this is not a weakness but shows true insight and courage. Take on too much and everything you do will suffer. If you can't look after yourself, how can you truly look after someone else?

Like the safety information on a plane, before you assist others always put your own oxygen mask on first, otherwise you could be sitting there for a long time starved of oxygen if you wait for other people to do this for you. Pay attention to your own needs and feelings so that you can be part of your loved-one's lives for as long as possible. Why not engage in activities that you enjoy and find relaxing as well as chauffeuring other people around to activities that they enjoy? Keep your body healthy by maintaining a balanced diet and exercising regularly. This will boost your confidence, mood and memory.

Look after yourself. Keep yourself well groomed; wash, trim, polish and moisturise regularly. Why not wear clothes that bring the best out in you? Remember that taking care of yourself means taking care of what is happening on the inside as well as the outside. Why not try something new such as yoga, tai chi, meditation, or mindfulness exercises? Do things that help you stay rooted in the *now*. Be calm and gently assertive when it comes to claiming your *me time*. Keep your mind and body primed to deal with the natural ups and downs in life.

5. Take charge of your happiness. If you want a better life you *can* make it happen! Just as you declutter your home, look at your life regularly and consider decluttering that as well. Learn to accept things that you cannot change. Consider the things you can change and ask yourself: 'Is it in my best interest to do so?'. If the answer is yes, then go about building a different life. Make a list of goals that are realistic and truly worth pursuing.

Try to keep things as simple as possible. For example, you don't need to slave away in the kitchen for hours every day, because a nutritionally balanced meal can be simple and quick to put together. Nor do you need to spend every minute of every day at work or rushing around trying to please everyone to the exclusion and detriment of yourself. Put time aside on a regular basis for your own development and the achievement of your own personal dreams and goals, even if it's just five minutes a day to start with. Give the mind a break from following all those compulsive thoughts. Remember that allowing the mind to run around untamed following thought after thought makes you unhappy. If things get too much, it is not good to suffer in silence; it is OK to speak up and ask for help.

A hobby can be an excellent way to carve out some dedicated time for yourself. Maybe there's something you've always wanted to do, such as learning to sketch, dance, or play a musical instrument. Maybe there's something you used to really enjoy that you've stopped doing. Joining a book club, local choir, charity or sports team may give you a new lease of life. It can give you the perfect excuse to break the monotony of the day and seize some time for yourself. In addition to giving you opportunities to make new friends and meet new 'radiators', a new hobby can help you feel motivated and exercise the 'grey matter'. It is a great way to take a break from a busy lifestyle and helps provide a sense of purpose. Engaging in enjoyable activities during *me time* helps to lower blood pressure and keep weight down.

Almost everyone has hang ups about themselves. For example, no matter how you look, there always seems to be some nagging body image issue. It is best to acknowledge and befriend these feelings. There comes a freedom with accepting your feelings and emotions as they are. They then lose their hold over you.

Smiling and keeping a positive orientation can help lift your mood by releasing certain hormones and chemicals in you as well as in those who see you smile. Neurotransmitters called endorphins are released when you smile. Endorphins make people feel happy, feel pain less, and reduce stress levels. They also dampen down the parts of your brain that are associated with worry and unhappiness. The level of the stress hormone, cortisol, also falls. So next time you are at work, at home, or on the way to lessons, smile. You will notice the world will gradually start to smile back. You will appear more approachable, and so interactions with people in your life will become smoother. It will make you a more appealing and attractive person to be around, which can only enhance your life at home and at work.[322,323]

It is your innate ability to be positive that is the key to changing yourself and your relationships. An optimistic outlook enables you to expect that good things will happen in your life and is associated with enjoying a longer life.[324] It is the positivity that comes through happiness which breeds success in life.

6. Self-discovery. Self-discovery can be defined as 'becoming aware of one's true potential, character and motives'. It means getting to know yourself better. What makes you 'tick'? What do you truly want? What is it that really inspires you? If you have no clear idea of who you are or what you want, how can you make life choices and decisions that are in your best interest? Unfortunately, not knowing yourself can result in a meaningless and unhappy life. It is important to realise what you want out of life. You need destinations, goals and aspirations, otherwise you may drift with no sense of purpose. Knowing yourself also helps you to keep healthy personal boundaries that enable you to feel empowered and protected.

Your life is essentially your journey of self-discovery and personal development. During the early years, you may have been conditioned to appear strong and resilient on the outside and to suppress any insecurities on the inside in an attempt to protect yourself from the world. At some point you are going to have to come to terms with, and accept and befriend, all that has been internalised. This internal spring-cleaning process can be nerve racking, but don't worry because you will emerge a more resilient and robust individual who is truer to him- or herself. It can help you develop insight and direction. It is time to drop any mask and start to be the person you truly are. This is not a sign of weakness; on the contrary, it takes strength, honesty and insight to achieve this. Once you understand and accept the stage that you are already at, life will give you what you need to develop further. It is time to open up, to trust in, and flow with life.

You often learn something about yourself as a result of a personal struggle or loss. The misfortune can test and then strengthen the 'metal' you are made of. Many people who have experienced tragedy and hardship have subsequently reported experiencing better relationships, a greater sense of self-worth, a renewed enthusiasm and a heightened appreciation for life. Even in the face of painful events, know that you *will* emerge as a stronger, more robust and resilient individual, so don't give into fear or worry. Never throw in the towel.

Make a list of your core values, such as empathy, compassion, honesty, love, kindness and loyalty. Then start to live and build your life around the core values that are important to you. Do not sacrifice or compromise them, regardless of what happens in your life. Stay true to yourself. Connect, stay rooted to, and develop, your internal strength and values.

Spend some time alone to get to know yourself better, whether meditating, practising mindfulness, reading, walking, or just being. Self-discovery is a process of gradual evolution to function at a higher frequency. You have the rest of your life to get to know yourself, so take your time, and always be gentle when looking at and assessing what is within.

Slowly and steadily start claiming and living the life you want to. Follow your true passions and purpose. For example, are you doing the job and following the career you truly want to follow, or are you trying to please someone else or live someone else's dreams? It is not material wealth that brings happiness; you cannot take your money with you, so why not do the things that you really want to do, even if it means having a little less cash in your pocket but having a fuller heart and a richer life? Money buys freedom from worry about the basics in life such as housing, food and clothes, but it does not buy happiness.[325]

It is time to stop being hard on yourself. You are here to experience life, develop and learn. It is OK to stumble, fall, get things wrong, because it is these very things that help us on our journey of self-discovery. Explore what life has to offer you, discover your true self, and start to live the life you truly want to.

7. Exploring life. Variety is the spice of life. Happiness with life can come from being curious and venturing beyond the boundaries of your comfort zone. When observing life, why see it just from one angle or perspective? Wouldn't you get bored with having exactly the same meal each day? If so, why not change things? Seeing and experiencing how other people perceive life teaches you a lot about yourself and your own stage of development, knowledge, tolerance and conditioning. Don't be afraid to try new healthy experiences or enjoy the diversity and vibrancy that life has to offer. Learn to gradually step out of your comfort zone. Try new healthy things that make you feel good, self-develop, and start to build that happier life.

People can start to feel as if they are stuck in a rut with the same day replaying over and over again. Nothing new or exciting appears to happen as life seems to lose some of its shine. People can end up sitting in the same place, eating the same food, having the same conversations, and rerunning the same mental frustrations and fantasies. You may start to dream of the same future moments of perceived magic that might release you from the seemingly mundane routine of everyday life. For example, you may start to imagine how they could spend the windfall from a large lottery win or find that one elusive relationship that would surely complete you and make everything in life OK. While dreaming in this way, people may begin to switch off and withdraw from the *present*, which deprives them of invaluable, fresh and new life experiences.[326,327]

Shaking things up and having fresh and varied experiences can be simpler to achieve than people imagine. Take a simple thing such as where you sit, whether at the dining table, in the lounge or at work. You may be surprised by how something as simple as sitting in a different place can change things. A different angle provides a different perspective on life. Sitting next to different people can change interactions and conversations. You start noticing things that may have completely passed you by before.

Individuals who experience well-being and happiness in life engage in a variety of activities. This can lead to an uplifting of mood and enhanced personal happiness. That feeling of the same old stuff tirelessly repeating is conquered. 'Mixing it up' is the key ingredient that prevents life from losing its impact and appeal.[328]

Why not think of something new, or an activity that you enjoyed in the past which you could try again, and actually go and do it? People often give up the things that they once enjoyed and which replenished them when the shroud of responsibility descends over them. It does not have to be this way. Take charge of your life and make a list of things that you would like to do, and, conversely, would like to drop from your life. Maybe start going for walks in the countryside, take up a previous passion, or try a new hobby, musical instrument, sporting activity, or even indulge in the occasional pampering session. Why not make your own list of wishes, wants, aspirations and dreams today? Here are a few suggestions that may help you. They require relatively little effort and cost. Maybe try one new activity a week? It might rekindle that innate human curiosity which too often gets dimmed along the path to adulthood.

- If possible, change the whole, or part of, the route you take to work.
- Go to an area with lots of restaurants and pick a place to eat where you have not thought to eat before.
- Go to the cinema and pick a random movie.
- Pick a place of interest near you that you have not been to and pay it a visit.
- Take time out to visit an old friend.
- Try new styles of food and drink.
- Go to the gym and work out with different machines, routines or classes.
- Go for a brisk walk or run on a route that you have not tried before.
- If you are single, ask someone out you have been mustering up the energy to ask, or consider joining a reputable dating agency.

Why not try something that involves joining a local group, maybe a new sport, or have a go at something that builds natural resilience, such as yoga, tai chi or meditative type practices? Meditation and spiritual practices can help people build connections, restore hope, improve mood and the ability to focus. They help develop that essential ability to be self-aware.

Maybe consider writing about your life experiences, keep a journal, or write a book; it is often said that everyone has a novel in them. The key is to identify what will work well for you as part of your own journey through life. No one knows you like you know yourself, so you are the one who is best placed to work this out. Always be vigilant about what you can change in your life and what will add flavour to it. For example, if there are aspects of your work you don't like, gradually move towards the work that you enjoy and let go of what is less rewarding for you as opportunities present themselves. Start engaging with things that play to your strengths and that revitalise and re-energise you. Why settle for second best?

8. Never, ever, give up! Once you have found yourself and identified what makes you happy and what you really want, take action. Set short-term, medium, and long-term goals, and never, ever give up in the pursuit of them. Once you've started, carry on moving forwards and don't look backwards. Say 'no' to doubt and fill yourself with positive affirmations. Things won't always go smoothly, but that is OK. If something is truly worth having and is life changing, the chances are it is going to take some hard work and perseverance to get there. Any obstacles that you overcome will make the fruits of your labour all the sweeter.

There will be setbacks, wrong turns and errors along the way, but that is OK. There will be doubters, obstacles and people who are unhelpful; forgive them. Remember that these are *your* dreams and not theirs. There is nothing that you cannot overcome when you truly put your mind, body and spirit behind it.

Focus on one task at a time. This is more effective than trying to achieve everything all in one go. Life is a marathon, not a sprint. It can be helpful to break down large tasks into smaller ones, and then bit by bit chip away at them. It is OK to ask for help when you need it from those you trust. The right amount of effort, action, concentration and dogged determination will get you over the finish line. Even when nobody else believes in you, keep believing in yourself because no one else knows you like you do.

9. The power of presence. It all boils down to the *here* and *now*, *this moment*, the only place where you can change, live your life and experience peace when you are ready to engage with life as it unfolds, rather than needlessly mind travelling to the past or future. Befriending *this moment* unconditionally, regardless of your life situation or what has happened, is something that anyone can master with practice.[178] Use your senses to stay rooted in what is happening within and without as you go about your daily tasks. Practising the art of staying *present* regardless of whether you are driving, washing the dishes or walking, is life changing. No matter how many times your attention gets distracted by your mind, keep bringing it back to the *now* without any self-criticism by watching or listening to something around you. If this becomes difficult or you feel internal tension, reconnect to your breathing. This is the way to tame a wandering mind and experience internal peace. Life will start to open up and become friendlier when you learn to befriend it and fully engage with it first in the only place you can, the *here* and *now*. Life has done its bit; it is patiently waiting for you to take this step. People who repeatedly mind-wander experience unhappiness, while those who have befriended the *now* live longer, are happier and have the best relationships.

Sometimes people think that the grass is greener on the other side of the fence. Frequently, however, on getting to the other side they find it is not. Happiness is also often projected into the future. If I have *x, y,* and not forgetting *z,* I will be happy, but this is not going to be the case. There is never a moment when it is not the *now*. If you become disengaged from the *present*, you miss the innate precious beauty of life.

The power of presence is what transcends your suffering and the life situations you find yourself in. Your happiness correlates directly with your ability to focus on what is happening *right now* in your life. It is living in the *now* that then correlates with the degree of well-being, health and success you experience, not your material possessions.

If you want good health, success and true change to come into your life, then change what is happening within you first. Start seeing things from a glass half full rather than a half-empty point of view. Be a 'radiator'. Start to see the positives rather than the constant negatives. Your happiness and life are in your hands. No one can or should be expected to make you happy; that is an unfair ask. Take charge! Make the *present moment* your constant companion as you travel through life and you will discover on taking this step that life tends to automatically unfold for the better.

Presence is the breeding ground for happiness and true change. Engage with each moment as it arises. See, feel, hear, smell and taste what is around you and within. Say *no* to lamenting about the past or becoming blinkered by worries about the future. In this way you can free yourself from all suffering. Start enjoying the peace, happiness and success that comes from the power of presence *right now* and say *no* to needless mind travel.

10. Me time. What makes you truly 'tick'? Once you have a clearer understanding of this, you will have a clearer understanding of what you truly want out of life and what *me time* really means for you. *Me time* can mean different things to people. It can encompass walking, reading, writing, cooking, exercising, meditating, praying, or just having five minutes alone with a hot drink and your feet up.

Make it a habit to put time for you regularly in your diary. Consider having a date night with yourself. Everyone needs to replenish themselves from time to time. It is important to make space to reflect on your life; where you are at, and where you'd like to be. Finding purpose in life increases satisfaction and well-being. *Me time* is not something to be aspired to; it is your basic need and right.

As well as sitting down for five minutes at home, realise other opportunities that may arise. Next time you are standing in a queue, take a few breaths and focus on what is around you, rather than worrying about what to cook for tea. If you like reading, keep a good book to hand so that when you are sitting in the car waiting to pick someone up you can read a few pages or switch off and listen to some relaxing music. Every time you get into your car or arrive somewhere, take a minute or so for yourself. While the lights are red, with your eyes open, take a few mindful breaths before you set off again. As well as packing healthy snacks for everyone else, why not keep a few for yourself. Regularly indulge in small pleasures, try new challenges, set and meet mini-goals, and maintain close social ties.

Have faith and believe in yourself. Stay upbeat, positive and keep on smiling, regardless of what is going on in the world. Make your happiness independent of what goes on outside and build it from the inside. Stay true to your core values, your sense of self, and do the best you can, fully charged and replenished.

If you want to be at your best for anyone in your life,
then first be the best you can be to yourself!

Chapter 14

A Perfect Reflection

Your life is a perfect reflection of what is going on inside you. No matter what steps are taken to conceal it, your inner state colours every aspect of your life. This includes your work, family, social and personal life. It influences your thoughts, moods, feelings and actions.

Any inner turmoil, negativity or resistance are the main obstacles to your happiness. When they are overcome, as you unconditionally accept and befriend what is happening within, only then can you experience peace. Only then can the external conditions of your life truly start to change for the better. People who are truly happy within are the genuine 'radiators' of warmth and positivity that arise from their core, and nourishes themselves and everyone around them. They give and receive freely, trusting in life. To be free, they let go of all that holds them back or weighs them down internally. At this level of functioning, life automatically opens up and becomes helpful. What was elusive before then seems much easier to achieve.

People who harbour bitterness and anguish tend to have fragmented social networks and unhappy life experiences. Inner change is the catalyst for outer change, not the other way around. Your life is what you make it. You are the architect of your own life! Only you have the ability to change yourself and transcend your life situations.

Befriend yourself just the way you are. Accept feelings, emotions, moods and thoughts for what they are, temporary and fleeting. If you stop struggling with them, they lose their hold over you. Start to engage with life as it unfolds, moment by moment rather than dwelling in the past or worrying about the future. As you become more *present*, you start to make the most of life's opportunities as they arise.

Carve out some regular *me time* so you can be fully charged to deal with anything life puts your way. In a busy, hectic life, try focusing on the one thing you are doing *right now*, regardless of how mundane or boring it is. Use everyday chores as practice material to stay connected to *this moment*. Look, hear, smell, feel and taste what is around you rather than be consumed by any negative compulsive thought patterns, moods or emotions. Stay *present*, focused and mindful on the interactions you are having with your partner and children, remembering that spending quality time with them is mutually beneficial to everyone. Unconditional love, support, and help, along with being mindful, helps the transition of any dependants to independence by letting them do what they can, as they are able to, while reinforcing healthy boundaries and equipping them with the tools necessary to succeed in life.

A sedentary lifestyle devoid of regular exercise and a balanced nutritional plan will also reflect on how long you live and the quality of life you enjoy. It will impact directly on your physical and mental well-being. But it is never too late to make a start on creating a healthier lifestyle. Sometimes people can lose their health in the process of trying to make every penny they can, only to spend every penny they've made trying to get their health back. Take charge of your life, because you are the only person who truly can. Keep yourself well hydrated, exercise regularly and eat a balanced diet containing fruits and vegetables, along with healthy proteins, carbohydrates and fats. Keep consumption of processed foods, unhealthy fats and simple sugars to a minimum. Treats are fine, but when they become the major or regular component of your dietary intake they only fuel poor health.

Why wait until your twilight years to live your dreams or tick off things on your bucket list? Start living the life you truly want *now*. Over the next few weeks consider writing a list of what you would truly like out of life – only you can figure out your aspirations and dreams. Why not spend the rest of your remaining days then living that life? Why not start ticking things off your bucket list as you go through life, rather than saving the best to last? Don't wait until the later stages of your life to rush to do what you really want to do because you may not be afforded enough, or, indeed, any time. Life can turn so easily like the ebb and flow of a tide.

All too often I see patients changing their lives only when they have had some form of wake-up call, such as a near death experience, an illness, or the loss of a loved one. It becomes the catalyst that changes them and their life. They became conscious of the adverse impact their lifestyle was having on their time in this world. They come to realise that there is no time like the *now* to start living the life they truly want to live.

A wake-up call often puts things into perspective and makes people take charge of their happiness. They stop worrying about the trivia and things they cannot change. Valuing what is really important starts to happen, along with filtering out of what isn't important. Material possessions stop becoming the be-all and end-all. A greater sense of gratitude, curiosity, purpose, compassion and empathy develops. As well as being more sociable, they start cultivating and nurturing the relationship with their true self, making some time for silence and solitude to develop self-awareness. *Me time* becomes a premium. Why wait for some trauma before you wake up and see the light? There is no time like *right now* to realise what actually and truly matters.

Be constantly mindful of how you speak to or treat people so that you don't have any cause for regret or suffering later. You never know when a conversation is going to be the last you have with a person, so choose your words wisely and speak your peace calmly. Having an air of open curiosity and putting yourself into somebody else's shoes helps you figure out why people behave the way they do. It is always better not to part with cross words.

Say no to negativity and yes to positivity. The mere repetition of positive words such as love, peace and compassion can turn on specific genes that lower physical and emotional stress. Positive people tend to feel better, live longer and have deeper and more trusting relationships, both at home and at work.[329,330] They become more in touch with their humanity, compassion, empathy and happiness, and enjoy a higher level of functioning.

As well as adding years to your life, why not add some life to your years? Stay positive and realise that you can overcome anything that life puts your way. Happiness is not a prize or a thing to be gained at some mystical future point; it is *here*, *right now*. The question really is: have you had enough of suffering in order to let go and embrace life in the only place possible? If so, say no to lamenting about the past, and no to worrying about the future. Start to embrace and join in with life in the only place you can, *this moment*.

It is never too late to change; nothing is fixed. You're never too old, too incumbent, or too burdened to do this. It is time to stop making excuses. Don't keep harping back to your past or blaming your conditioning, parenting, broken relationships, colleagues or family for your unhappiness. Your happiness is where it has always been, in your own hands. No one has had a perfect life. It is the challenges and traumas of life that fuel personal growth and the development to a stronger level of grit, robustness and resilience. Start to see the challenges that test you as opportunities to move to higher levels of functioning and development which will eventually free you from all negativity, suffering and needless mind-wandering.

The only person who can truly bring change to your life is you. It has always been that way. No one can make you happy: only you can do this. It is time for you to look after yourself, in addition to your responsibilities. Life is not about self-sacrifice. Armed with adequate *me time*, you can achieve a balance between what you need to do, and practice self-growth and self-preservation, no matter who you are or what your life situation is.

Me time is essential if you want to be at your best for yourself and the people you care about. It is not being selfish; it is ensuring that you are in prime physical and mental health to perform at your very best. You can lead by example and show those around you how they too can have thriving, happiness and success in a frantic modern-day world, even when faced with adversity. Become the world you want to see. Start living the life you truly want and deserve. Inner change is the catalyst for outer change. Your happiness is what breeds success in love and life. Happiness is not something you can find outside of yourself. You cannot earn your way to it; you can only realise that it exists within you already, and unconditionally befriend it. It is your basic human right to have time to eat well, exercise, replenish, recuperate, enjoy, live, laugh and love in life!

Everyone has a basic right to have me time. That includes you!
So, start carving some me time out for yourself,
and for loving yourself just the way you are.
After all, you are the most important relationship you will ever have.
You are unique in the whole of the universe.
Never before has there ever been anyone like you.
What could be more beautiful than that?

Abbreviations

BMI   Body Mass Index
BMR   Basal Metabolic Rate
BPD   Borderline personality disorder
CASH   Consensus Action on Salt and Health
CBT   Cognitive-behavioural therapy
DBT   Dialectical-behaviour therapy
EFA   Essential fatty acid
ERD   Emotional regulation disorder
FODMAP Fermentable Oligosaccharides, Disaccharides, Monosaccharides and Polyols
g   Grams
HDL   High-density lipoproteins
HIIT   High Intensity Interval Training
h/d   Hours per day
IBD   Inflammatory Bowel Disease
IBS   Irritable bowel syndrome
l/d   Litres per day
Kcal/d Kilocalories used per day
Kg   Kilograms
LDL   Low-density lipoproteins
MBCT   Mindfulness-based cognitive therapy
MICT   Moderate-intensity continuous training
mg   Milligrams
min/wk Minutes per week
NICE   National Institute for Health and Care Excellence
PSHE   Personal social and health education
USDA   U.S. Department of Agriculture
WHO   World Health Organisation

References

1. Oxford, D. balance - definition of balance in English. *https://en.oxforddictionaries.com/definition/balance*
2. Charness, G. & Dufwenberg, M. Promises and Partnership. *Econometrica* **74,** 1579–1601 (2006).
3. Reeves, W. C. *et al.* Mental illness surveillance among adults in the United States. *MMWR Surveill. Summ.* **60,** 1–29 (2011).
4. Myers, D. G. The funds, friends, and faith of happy people. *Am. Psychol.* **55,** 56–67 (2000).
5. Easterlin, R. A., McVey, L. A., Switek, M., Sawangfa, O. & Zweig, J. S. The happiness–income paradox revisited. *Proc. Natl. Acad. Sci. U. S. A.* **107,** 22463–22468 (2010).
6. Maslach, C. *Burnout: The cost of caring.* (ISHK, 2003).
7. Maslach, C. & Jackson, S. E. The measurement of experienced burnout. *J. Organ. Behav.* **2,** 99–113 (1981).
8. Maslach, C. & Leiter, M. P. Early predictors of job burnout and engagement. *J. Appl. Psychol.* **93,** 498–512 (2008).
9. GBD 2013 Risk Factors Collaborators *et al.* Global, regional, and national comparative risk assessment of 79 behavioural, environmental and occupational, and metabolic risks or clusters of risks in 188 countries, 1990-2013: a systematic analysis for the Global Burden of Disease Study 2013. *Lancet* **386,** 2287–2323 (2015).
10. Elvsåshagen, T. *et al.* The load of short telomeres is increased and associated with lifetime number of depressive episodes in bipolar II disorder. *J. Affect. Disord.* **135,** 43–50 (2011).
11. Farrag, W., Eid, M., El-Shazly, S. & Abdallah, M. Angiotensin II type 1 receptor gene polymorphism and telomere shortening in essential hypertension. *Mol. Cell. Biochem.* **351,** 13–18 (2011).
12. Ogami, M. *et al.* Telomere shortening in human coronary artery diseases. *Arterioscler. Thromb. Vasc. Biol.* **24,** 546–550 (2004).
13. Yamada, N. Telomere shortening, atherosclerosis, and metabolic syndrome. *Intern. Med.* **42,** 135–136 (2003).
14. Lovasz, B. D., Golovics, P. A., Vegh, Z. & Lakatos, P. L. New trends in inflammatory bowel disease epidemiology and disease course in Eastern Europe. *Dig. Liver Dis.* **45,** 269–276 (2013).
15. Oyebode, O., Gordon-Dseagu, V., Walker, A. & Mindell, J. S. Fruit and vegetable consumption and all-cause, cancer and CVD mortality: analysis of Health Survey for England data. *J. Epidemiol. Community Health* jech–2013–203500 (2014).
16. Clemente, J. C., Ursell, L. K., Parfrey, L. W. & Knight, R. The impact of the gut microbiota on human health: an integrative view. *Cell* **148,** 1258–1270 (2012).
17. Van Praag, H., Kempermann, G. & Gage, F. H. Running increases cell proliferation and neurogenesis in the adult mouse dentate gyrus. *Nat. Neurosci.* **2,** 266–270 (1999).
18. Draganski, B. *et al.* Temporal and spatial dynamics of brain structure changes during extensive learning. *J. Neurosci.* **26,** 6314–6317 (2006).
19. Colcombe, S. J. *et al.* Aerobic exercise training increases brain volume in aging

humans. *J. Gerontol. A Biol. Sci. Med. Sci.* **61,** 1166–1170 (2006).
20. Aune, D. *et al.* Whole grain consumption and risk of cardiovascular disease, cancer, and all cause and cause specific mortality: systematic review and dose-response meta-analysis of prospective studies. *BMJ* **353,** i2716 (2016).
21. Diet, nutrition and the prevention of chronic diseases. *World Health Organ. Tech. Rep. Ser.* **916,** i–viii, 1–149, backcover (2003).
22. Cheuvront, S. N. & Kenefick, R. W. Dehydration: physiology, assessment, and performance effects. *Compr. Physiol.* **4,** 257–285 (2014).
23. Nicolaidis, S. Physiology of thirst. *Hydration Throughout Life* 3–8 (1998).
24. Choices, N. Six to eight glasses of water 'still best'. *NHS choices* Available at: www.nhs.uk/news/food-and-diet/six-to-eight-glasses-of-water-still-best/ps. (Accessed: 25th October 2017)
25. Heller, K. E., Sohn, W., Burt, B. A. & Eklund, S. A. Water consumption in the United States in 1994--96 and implications for water fluoridation policy. *J. Public Health Dent.* **59,** 3–11 (1999).
26. Taivainen, H., Laitinen, K., Tähtelä, R., Kilanmaa, K. & Välimäki, M. J. Role of plasma vasopressin in changes of water balance accompanying acute alcohol intoxication. *Alcohol. Clin. Exp. Res.* **19,** 759–762 (1995).
27. Maughan, R. J. & Griffin, J. Caffeine ingestion and fluid balance: a review. *J. Hum. Nutr. Diet.* **16,** 411–420 (2003).
28. Coffee Statistics - Coffee Facts, Coffee Industry Stats. Available at: http://www.coffee-statistics.com. (Accessed: 26th October 2017)
29. European Food Safety Authority. Caffeine: EFSA consults on draft assessment. (2015). Available at: http://www.efsa.europa.eu/en/press/news/150115. (Accessed: 12th July 2016)
30. Greden, J. F. Anxiety or caffeinism: a diagnostic dilemma. *Am. J. Psychiatry* **131,** 1089–1092 (1974).
31. Cohen, S. Pathogenesis of coffee-induced gastrointestinal symptoms. *N. Engl. J. Med.* **303,** 122–124 (1980).
32. Sigmon, S. C., Herning, R. I., Better, W., Cadet, J. L. & Griffiths, R. R. Caffeine withdrawal, acute effects, tolerance, and absence of net beneficial effects of chronic administration: cerebral blood flow velocity, quantitative EEG, and subjective effects. *Psychopharmacology* **204,** 573–585 (2009).
33. Beetz, R. Mild dehydration: a risk factor of urinary tract infection? *Eur. J. Clin. Nutr.* **57 Suppl 2,** S52–8 (2003).
34. Atan, L. *et al.* High kidney stone risk in men working in steel industry at hot temperatures. *Urology* **65,** 858–861 (2005).
35. Mentes, J. Oral hydration in older adults: greater awareness is needed in preventing, recognizing, and treating dehydration. *Am. J. Nurs.* **106,** 40–9; (2006).
36. Ellis, K. J. Human body composition: in vivo methods. *Physiol. Rev.* **80,** 649–680 (2000).
37. D'Anci, K. E., Mahoney, C. R., Vibhakar, A., Kanter, J. H. & Taylor, H. A. Voluntary Dehydration and Cognitive Performance in Trained College Athletes. *Percept. Mot. Skills* **109,** 251–269 (2009).
38. Cian, C., Barraud, P. A., Melin, B. & Raphel, C. Effects of fluid ingestion on cognitive function after heat stress or exercise-induced dehydration. *Int. J. Psychophysiol.* **42,** 243–251 (2001).
39. Institute of Medicine (us) Panel on Dietary Reference Intakes & Water. *DRI, dietary reference intakes for water, potassium, sodium, chloride, and sulfate.* (National

Academy Press, 2005).

40. Agostoni, C. V., Bresson, J. L., Fairweather-Tait, S. & Others. Scientific opinion on dietary reference values for water. *EFSA J* **8,** (2010).

41. Valtin, H. & Others. 'Drink at least eight glasses of water a day.' Really? Is there scientific evidence for '8× 8'? *American Journal of Physiology-Regulatory, Integrative and Comparative Physiology* **283,** R993–R1004 (2002).

42. Adolph, E. F. Physiological regulations. (1943). doi:10.5962/bhl.title.6393

43. Armstrong, L. E., Costill, D. L. & Fink, W. J. Influence of diuretic-induced dehydration on competitive running performance. *Med. Sci. Sports Exerc.* **17,** 456–461 (1985).

44. Maughan, R. J. Impact of mild dehydration on wellness and on exercise performance. *Eur. J. Clin. Nutr.* **57,** S19–S23 (2003).

45. Shirreffs, S. M., Armstrong, L. E. & Cheuvront, S. N. Fluid and electrolyte needs for preparation and recovery from training and competition. *J. Sports Sci.* **22,** 57–63 (2004).

46. Gutmann, F. D. & Gardner, J. W. Fatal water intoxication of an Army trainee during urine drug testing. *Mil. Med.* **167,** 435–437 (2002).

47. Lindeman, R. D., Van Buren, H. C. & Raisz, L. G. Osmolar renal concentrating ability in healthy young men and hospitalized patients without renal disease. *N. Engl. J. Med.* **262,** 1306–1309 (1960).

48. Sawka, M. N., Cheuvront, S. N. & Carter, R., 3rd. Human water needs. *Nutr. Rev.* **63,** S30–9 (2005).

49. Hayes, P. A., Fraher, M. H. & Quigley, E. M. M. Irritable bowel syndrome: the role of food in pathogenesis and management. *Gastroenterol. Hepatol.* **10,** 164–174 (2014).

50. Moynihan, P. J. & Kelly, S. A. M. Effect on caries of restricting sugars intake: systematic review to inform WHO guidelines. *J. Dent. Res.* **93,** 8–18 (2014).

51. Johnson, R. K. *et al.* Dietary sugars intake and cardiovascular health: a scientific statement from the American Heart Association. *Circulation* **120,** 1011–1020 (2009).

52. WHO. WHO urges global action to curtail consumption and health impacts of sugary drinks. *who* (2016). Available at: http://www.who.int/mediacentre/news/releases/2016/curtail-sugary-drinks/en/. (Accessed: 12th June 2016)

53. MacGregor, G. A. & Hashem, K. M. Action on sugar—lessons from UK salt reduction programme. *Lancet* **383,** 929–931 (2014).

54. Kelly, T., Yang, W., Chen, C.-S., Reynolds, K. & He, J. Global burden of obesity in 2005 and projections to 2030. *Int. J. Obes.* **32,** 1431–1437 (2008).

55. Wyness, L. A., Butriss, J. L. & Stanner, S. A. Reducing the population's sodium intake: the UK Food Standards Agency's salt reduction programme. *Public Health Nutr.* **15,** 254–261 (2012).

56. Ha, S. K. Dietary salt intake and hypertension. *Electrolyte Blood Press.* **12,** 7–18 (2014).

57. Wang, X.-Q., Terry, P.-D. & Yan, H. Review of salt consumption and stomach cancer risk: epidemiological and biological evidence. *World J. Gastroenterol.* **15,** 2204–2213 (2009).

58. Sutherland, J., Edwards, P., Shankar, B. & Dangour, A. D. Fewer adults add salt at the table after initiation of a national salt campaign in the UK: a repeated cross-sectional analysis. *Br. J. Nutr.* **110,** 552–558 (2013).

59. Seery, S. & Jakeman, P. A metered intake of milk following exercise and thermal dehydration restores whole-body net fluid balance better than a carbohydrate–electrolyte solution or water in healthy young men. *Br. J. Nutr.* **116,** 1013–1021 (2016).

60. Bredenoord, A. J., Weusten, B. L. A. M., Sifrim, D., Timmer, R. & Smout, A. J. P. M. Aerophagia, gastric, and supragastric belching: a study using intraluminal electrical impedance monitoring. *Gut* **53,** 1561–1565 (2004).

61. McNab, B. K. On the utility of uniformity in the definition of basal rate of metabolism. *Physiol. Zool.* **70,** 718–720 (1997).

62. Elia, M., Ritz, P. & Stubbs, R. J. Total energy expenditure in the elderly. *Eur. J. Clin. Nutr.* **54 Suppl 3,** S92–103 (2000).

63. McMurray, R. G., Soares, J., Caspersen, C. J. & McCurdy, T. Examining variations of resting metabolic rate of adults: a public health perspective. *Med. Sci. Sports Exerc.* **46,** 1352–1358 (2014).

64. van Aggel-Leijssen, D. P., Saris, W. H., Hul, G. B. & van Baak, M. A. Short-term effects of weight loss with or without low-intensity exercise training on fat metabolism in obese men. *Am. J. Clin. Nutr.* **73,** 523–531 (2001).

65. Hsu, T. M. *et al.* Hippocampus ghrelin signaling mediates appetite through lateral hypothalamic orexin pathways. *Elife* **4,** (2015).

66. Plachta-Danielzik, S. *et al.* Energy Gain and Energy Gap in Normal-weight Children: Longitudinal Data of the KOPS. *Obesity* **16,** 777–783 (2008).

67. Zhai, F., Wang, H., Wang, Z., Popkin, B. M. & Chen, C. Closing the energy gap to prevent weight gain in China. *Obes. Rev.* **9 Suppl 1,** 107–112 (2008).

68. NHS. What should my daily intake of calories be? *NHS Choices* Available at: http://www.nhs.uk/chq/pages/1126.aspx?categoryid=51&subcategoryid=165). (Accessed: 12th July 2016)

69. Government, A. & National Health and Medical Research Council. Nutrient Reference Values. *nrv.gov.au* (updated 24.11.2016). Available at: https://www.nrv.gov.au/dietary-energy. (Accessed: 12th December 2016)

70. Clinic, M. Daily calorie intake calculator. *Mayo Clinic* Available at: www.mayoclinic.org/healthy-lifestyle/weight-loss/in-depth/weight-loss/itt-20084941. (Accessed: 25th October 2017)

71. Gray, A. Nutritional Recommendations for Individuals with Diabetes. in *Endotext* (eds. De Groot, L. J. et al.) (MDText.com, Inc., 2015).

72. Pollard, C. M., Miller, M. R. & Daly, A. M. Increasing fruit and vegetable consumption: success of the Western Australian Go for 2&5® campaign. *Public Health* (2008).

73. Aune, D. *et al.* Fruit and vegetable intake and the risk of cardiovascular disease, total cancer and all-cause mortality-a systematic review and dose-response meta-analysis of prospective studies. *Int. J. Epidemiol.* **46,** 1029–1056 (2017).

74. Fuentes-Zaragoza, E., Riquelme-Navarrete, M. J., Sánchez-Zapata, E. & Pérez-Álvarez, J. A. Resistant starch as functional ingredient: A review. *Food Res. Int.* **43,** 931–942 (2010/5).

75. Shepherd, S. J., Lomer, M. C. E. & Gibson, P. R. Short-chain carbohydrates and functional gastrointestinal disorders. *Am. J. Gastroenterol.* **108,** 707–717 (2013).

76. Spiegel, B. M. R. The burden of IBS: looking at metrics. *Curr. Gastroenterol. Rep.* **11,** 265–269 (2009).

77. Spiller, R. *et al.* Guidelines on the irritable bowel syndrome: mechanisms and practical management. *Gut* **56,** 1770–1798 (2007).

78. NICE. Irritable bowel syndrome and diet. *NICE Guidelines* Available at: http://www.unimed.co.uk/website/G81071/files/Irritable_Bowel_Syndrome.p df. (Accessed: 2nd February 2017)

79. Wang, X. *et al.* Fruit and vegetable consumption and mortality from all causes, cardiovascular disease, and cancer: systematic review and dose-response meta-analysis of prospective cohort studies. *BMJ* **349,** g4490 (2014).

80. Carbohydrate reference list. *www.diabetes.org.uk.*

81. American Diabetes Association. Nutrition Recommendations and Interventions for Diabetes. *Diabetes Care* **30,** S48–S65 (2007).

82. King, J. C. & Slavin, J. L. White potatoes, human health, and dietary guidance. *Adv. Nutr.* **4,** 393S–401S (2013).

83. Camire, M. E., Kubow, S. & Donnelly, D. J. Potatoes and human health. *Crit. Rev. Food Sci. Nutr.* **49,** 823–840 (2009).

84. Quamruzzaman, M. Resistant starch a new weapon against disease fighting of potato eater: A focused review. *Asian Journal of Pharmaceutics* **10,** 01–05 (2016).

85. Lomer, M. C. E. Review article: the aetiology, diagnosis, mechanisms and clinical evidence for food intolerance. *Aliment. Pharmacol. Ther.* **41,** 262–275 (2015).

86. Lever, E., Cole, J., Scott, S. M., Emery, P. W. & Whelan, K. Systematic review: the effect of prunes on gastrointestinal function. *Aliment. Pharmacol. Ther.* **40,** 750–758 (2014).

87. Harrington, A. M. *et al.* A novel role for TRPM8 in visceral afferent function. *Pain* **152,** 1459–1468 (2011).

88. University, M. Low FODMAP diet for Irritable Bowel Syndrome. *monash.ed* Available at: http://www.med.monash.edu/cecs/gastro/fodmap/. (Accessed: 19th December 2016)

89. Fernández-Bañares, F. *et al.* Sugar malabsorption in functional abdominal bloating: a pilot study on the long-term effect of dietary treatment. *Clin. Nutr.* **25,** 824–831 (2006).

90. Gujral, N., Freeman, H. J. & Thomson, A. B. R. Celiac disease: prevalence, diagnosis, pathogenesis and treatment. *World J. Gastroenterol.* **18,** 6036–6059 (2012).

91. Biesiekierski, J. R. *et al.* Gluten causes gastrointestinal symptoms in subjects without celiac disease: a double-blind randomized placebo-controlled trial. *Am. J. Gastroenterol.* **106,** 508–14; quiz 515 (2011).

92. Lebwohl, B. *et al.* Long term gluten consumption in adults without celiac disease and risk of coronary heart disease: prospective cohort study. *BMJ* **357,** j1892 (2017).

93. Wu, G. Dietary protein intake and human health. *Food Funct.* **7,** 1251–1265 (2016).

94. Micha, R., Wallace, S. K. & Mozaffarian, D. Red and processed meat consumption and risk of incident coronary heart disease, stroke, and diabetes mellitus a systematic review and meta-analysis. *Circulation* (2010).

95. Larsson, S. C. & Wolk, A. Meat consumption and risk of colorectal cancer: a meta-analysis of prospective studies. *International journal of cancer* (2006).

96. Nilsen, R., Høstmark, A. T., Haug, A. & Skeie, S. Effect of a high intake of cheese on cholesterol and metabolic syndrome: results of a randomized trial. *Food Nutr. Res.* **59,** 27651 (2015).

97. Pan, A., Sun, Q. & Bernstein, A. M. Red meat consumption and mortality: results from 2 prospective cohort studies. *Archives of* (2012).

98. Zheng, J. *et al.* Fish consumption and CHD mortality: an updated meta-analysis of seventeen cohort studies. *Public Health Nutr.* **15,** 725–737 (2012).

99. Chowdhury, R. *et al.* Association between fish consumption, long chain omega 3 fatty acids, and risk of cerebrovascular disease: systematic review and meta-analysis. *BMJ* **345,** e6698 (2012).

100. Virtanen, J. K., Mozaffarian, D., Chiuve, S. E. & Rimm, E. B. Fish consumption and risk of major chronic disease in men. *Am. J. Clin. Nutr.* **88,** 1618–1625 (2008).

101. Morris, M. C., Evans, D. A., Tangney, C. C., Bienias, J. L. & Wilson, R. S. Fish consumption and cognitive decline with age in a large community study. *Arch. Neurol.* **62,** 1849–1853 (2005).

102. Craig, W. J. & Mangels, A. R. Position of the American Dietetic Association: vegetarian diets. *J. Am. Diet. Assoc.* (2009).

103. Pesta, D. H. & Samuel, V. T. A high-protein diet for reducing body fat: mechanisms and possible caveats. *Nutr. Metab.* **11,** 53 (2014).

104. Westerterp-Plantenga, M. S., Lejeune, M. P. G. M., Nijs, I., van Ooijen, M. & Kovacs, E. M. R. High protein intake sustains weight maintenance after body weight loss in humans. *Int. J. Obes. Relat. Metab. Disord.* **28,** 57–64 (2004).

105. Walker, C. & Reamy, B. V. Diets for cardiovascular disease prevention: what is the evidence? *Am. Fam. Physician* **79,** 571–578 (2009).

106. Andersson, A. & Bryngelsson, S. Towards a healthy diet: from nutrition recommendations to dietary advice. *Scandinavian Journal of Food & Nutrition* **51,** 31 (2007).

107. USDA. Estimated Calorie Needs per Day, by Age, Sex, and Physical Activity Level. (2015). Available at: http://health.gov/dietaryguidelines/2015/guidelines/appendix-2/. (Accessed: 12th July 2016)

108. Mettler, S., Mitchell, N. & Tipton, K. D. Increased protein intake reduces lean body mass loss during weight loss in athletes. *Med. Sci. Sports Exerc.* **42,** 326–337 (2010).

109. Phillips, S. M. & Van Loon, L. J. C. Dietary protein for athletes: from requirements to optimum adaptation. *J. Sports Sci.* **29 Suppl 1,** S29–38 (2011).

110. Barzel, U. S. & Massey, L. K. Excess Dietary Protein Can Adversely Affect Bone. *J. Nutr.* **128,** 1051–1053 (1998).

111. Hooper, L. *et al.* Reduced or modified dietary fat for preventing cardiovascular disease. *Cochrane Database Syst. Rev.* CD002137 (2011).

112. Qin, J. *et al.* A human gut microbial gene catalogue established by metagenomic sequencing. *Nature* **464,** 59–65 (2010).

113. Sender, R., Fuchs, S. & Milo, R. Revised Estimates for the Number of Human and Bacteria Cells in the Body. *PLoS Biol.* **14,** e1002533 (2016).

114. O'Hara, A. M. & Shanahan, F. The gut flora as a forgotten organ. *EMBO Rep.* **7,** 688–693 (2006).

115. Guglielmetti, S., Mora, D., Gschwender, M. & Popp, K. Randomised clinical trial: Bifidobacterium bifidum MIMBb75 significantly alleviates irritable bowel syndrome and improves quality of life----a double-blind, placebo-controlled study. *Aliment. Pharmacol. Ther.* **33,** 1123–1132 (2011).

116. Fortmann, S. P., Burda, B. U., Senger, C. A., Lin, J. S. & Whitlock, E. P. Vitamin and mineral supplements in the primary prevention of cardiovascular disease and cancer: an updated systematic evidence review for the US

Preventive Services Task Force. *Ann. Intern. Med.* **159,** 824–834 (2013).

117. Doll, R., Peto, R., Wheatley, K., Gray, R. & Sutherland, I. Mortality in relation to smoking: 40 years' observations on male British doctors. *BMJ* **309,** 901–911 (1994).

118. Doll, R., Peto, R., Boreham, J. & Sutherland, I. Mortality in relation to smoking: 50 years' observations on male British doctors. *BMJ* **328,** 1519 (2004).

119. Saha, S. P., Bhalla, D. K., Whayne, T. F., Jr & Gairola, C. Cigarette smoke and adverse health effects: An overview of research trends and future needs. *Int. J. Angiol.* **16,** 77–83 (2007).

120. Sinn, D. H. *et al.* The speed of eating and functional dyspepsia in young women. *Gut Liver* **4,** 173–178 (2010).

121. Maruyama, K. *et al.* The joint impact on being overweight of self-reported behaviours of eating quickly and eating until full: cross sectional survey. *BMJ* **337,** a2002 (2008).

122. Tolle, V. *et al.* Ultradian rhythmicity of ghrelin secretion in relation with GH, feeding behavior, and sleep-wake patterns in rats. *Endocrinology* **143,** 1353–1361 (2002).

123. Williams, J. & Mobarhan, S. A critical interaction: leptin and ghrelin. *Nutr. Rev.* **61,** 391–393 (2003).

124. Birch, L., Savage, J. S. & Ventura, A. Influences on the Development of Children's Eating Behaviours: From Infancy to Adolescence. *Can. J. Diet. Pract. Res.* **68,** s1–s56 (2007).

125. Sheeran, P., Gollwitzer, P. M. & Bargh, J. A. Nonconscious processes and health. *Health Psychol.* **32,** 460–473 (2013).

126. Cools, J., Schotte, D. E. & McNally, R. J. Emotional arousal and overeating in restrained eaters. *J. Abnorm. Psychol.* **101,** 348–351 (1992).

127. Adam, T. C. & Epel, E. S. Stress, eating and the reward system. *Physiol. Behav.* **91,** 449–458 (2007).

128. Hudson, J. I., Hiripi, E., Pope, H. G., Jr & Kessler, R. C. The prevalence and correlates of eating disorders in the National Comorbidity Survey Replication. *Biol. Psychiatry* **61,** 348–358 (2007).

129. O'Reilly, G. A., Cook, L., Spruijt-Metz, D. & Black, D. S. Mindfulness-based interventions for obesity-related eating behaviours: a literature review. *Obes. Rev.* **15,** 453–461 (2014).

130. Kabat-Zinn, J. *Wherever You Go, There You Are: Mindfulness Meditation In Everyday Life.* (Hachette UK, 2009).

131. Schroevers, M. J. & Brandsma, R. Is learning mindfulness associated with improved affect after mindfulness-based cognitive therapy? *Br. J. Psychol.* **101,** 95–107 (2010).

132. Wansink, B. From mindless eating to mindlessly eating better. *Physiol. Behav.* **100,** 454–463 (2010).

133. Arch, J. J. *et al.* Enjoying food without caloric cost: The impact of brief mindfulness on laboratory eating outcomes. *Behav. Res. Ther.* **79,** 23–34 (2016).

134. Killingsworth, M. A. & Gilbert, D. T. A wandering mind is an unhappy mind. *Science* **330,** 932 (2010).

135. Moore, S. C. *et al.* Leisure time physical activity of moderate to vigorous intensity and mortality: a large pooled cohort analysis. *PLoS Med.* **9,** e1001335 (2012).

136. Lee, I.-M. *et al.* Effect of physical inactivity on major non-communicable

diseases worldwide: an analysis of burden of disease and life expectancy. *Lancet* **380,** 219–229 (2012).

137. Tremblay, M. S. *et al.* Systematic review of sedentary behaviour and health indicators in school-aged children and youth. *Int. J. Behav. Nutr. Phys. Act.* **8,** 98 (2011).

138. Foundation, B. H. Are you sitting too much? *British Heart Foundation* Available at: https://www.bhf.org.uk/heart-matters-magazine/activity/sitting-down. (Accessed: 1st June 2017)

139. Colcombe, S. J. *et al.* Aerobic fitness reduces brain tissue loss in aging humans. *J. Gerontol. A Biol. Sci. Med. Sci.* **58,** 176–180 (2003).

140. Ishihara, T., Sugasawa, S., Matsuda, Y. & Mizuno, M. Improved executive functions in 6-12-year-old children following cognitively engaging tennis lessons. *J. Sports Sci.* 1–7 (2016).

141. Hallgren, M. *et al.* Exercise and internet-based cognitive-behavioural therapy for depression: multicentre randomised controlled trial with 12-month follow-up. *Br. J. Psychiatry* **209,** 414–420 (2016).

142. Garber, C. E. *et al.* American College of Sports Medicine position stand. Quantity and quality of exercise for developing and maintaining cardiorespiratory, musculoskeletal, and neuromotor fitness in apparently healthy adults: guidance for prescribing exercise. *Med. Sci. Sports Exerc.* **43,** 1334–1359 (2011).

143. NHS. Fitness. *NHS UK Live Well* Available at: www.nhs.uk/LiveWell/Fitness/Pages/Fitnesshome.aspx. (Accessed: 25th October 2017)

144. Emberts, T., Porcari, J., Dobers-Tein, S., Steffen, J. & Foster, C. Exercise intensity and energy expenditure of a tabata workout. *J. Sports Sci. Med.* **12,** 612–613 (2013).

145. Foster, C. *et al.* The Effects of High Intensity Interval Training vs Steady State Training on Aerobic and Anaerobic Capacity. *J. Sports Sci. Med.* **14,** 747–755 (2015).

146. Ross, A. & Thomas, S. The health benefits of yoga and exercise: a review of comparison studies. *J. Altern. Complement. Med.* **16,** 3–12 (2010).

147. Balasubramaniam, M., Telles, S. & Doraiswamy, P. M. Yoga on our minds: a systematic review of yoga for neuropsychiatric disorders. *Front. Psychiatry* **3,** 117 (2012).

148. Khalsa, S. B. S., Shorter, S. M., Cope, S., Wyshak, G. & Sklar, E. Yoga ameliorates performance anxiety and mood disturbance in young professional musicians. *Appl. Psychophysiol. Biofeedback* **34,** 279–289 (2009).

149. Streeter, C. C. *et al.* Effects of yoga versus walking on mood, anxiety, and brain GABA levels: a randomized controlled MRS study. *J. Altern. Complement. Med.* **16,** 1145–1152 (2010).

150. Sherman, K. J., Cherkin, D. C., Erro, J., Miglioretti, D. L. & Deyo, R. A. Comparing yoga, exercise, and a self-care book for chronic low back pain: a randomized, controlled trial. *Ann. Intern. Med.* **143,** 849–856 (2005).

151. Yoga could be good for heart disease. Simultaneous focus on body, breathing, and mind may be just what the doctor ordered. *Harv. Heart Lett.* **21,** 5 (2010).

152. Jahnke, R., Larkey, L., Rogers, C., Etnier, J. & Lin, F. A comprehensive review of health benefits of qigong and tai chi. *Am. J. Health Promot.* **24,** e1–e25 (2010).

153. Lee, M. S. & Ernst, E. Systematic reviews of t'ai chi: an overview. *Br. J. Sports*

Med. **46,** 713–718 (2012).

154. Abbott, R. & Lavretsky, H. Tai Chi and Qigong for the treatment and prevention of mental disorders. *Psychiatr. Clin. North Am.* **36,** 109–119 (2013).

155. Hölzel, B. K. *et al.* Mindfulness practice leads to increases in regional brain gray matter density. *Psychiatry Res.* **191,** 36–43 (2011).

156. Lazar, S. W. *et al.* Functional brain mapping of the relaxation response and meditation. *Neuroreport* **11,** 1581–1585 (2000).

157. Epel, E. S. *et al.* Accelerated telomere shortening in response to life stress. *Proc. Natl. Acad. Sci. U. S. A.* **101,** 17312–17315 (2004).

158. Diener, E. & Chan, M. Y. Happy people live longer: Subjective well-being contributes to health and longevity. *Appl. Psychol. Health Well Being* **3,** 1–43 (2011).

159. Wiest, M., Schüz, B., Webster, N. & Wurm, S. Subjective well-being and mortality revisited: differential effects of cognitive and emotional facets of well-being on mortality. *Health Psychol.* **30,** 728–735 (2011).

160. Lundberg, U. Stress hormones in health and illness: the roles of work and gender. *Psychoneuroendocrinology* **30,** 1017–1021 (2005).

161. World Health Organization. 1.1 billion people at risk of hearing loss; 2015. *World Health Organization* (2015). Available at: http://www.who.int/pbd/deafness/activities/MLS_Brochure_English_lowres _for_web.pdf. (Accessed: March 2018)

162. Hilbert, M. & López, P. The world's technological capacity to store, communicate, and compute information. *Science* **332,** 60–65 (2011).

163. cbsnews.com/news. phantom-vibration-syndrome-common-in-cellphone-users. (2016). Available at: https://www.cbsnews.com/news/phantom-vibration-syndrome-common-in-cellphone-users/. (Accessed: 11th January 2017)

164. Rothberg, M. B. *et al.* Phantom vibration syndrome among medical staff: a cross sectional survey. *BMJ* **341,** c6914 (2010).

165. Kuchinskas, S. *The Chemistry of Connection: How the Oxytocin Response Can Help You Find Trust, Intimacy, and Love.* (New Harbinger Publications, 2009).

166. Alter, A. *Irresistible: The rise of addictive technology and the business of keeping us hooked.* (Penguin, 2017).

167. Eddy, R. Sleep deprivation among physicians. *B. C. Med. J.* **47,** 176 (2005).

168. Miller, N. L., Matsangas, P. & Shattuck, L. G. Fatigue and its effect on performance in military environments. *Performance under stress* **2007,** 231–249 (2008).

169. Hartzler, B. M. Fatigue on the flight deck: the consequences of sleep loss and the benefits of napping. *Accid. Anal. Prev.* **62,** 309–318 (2014).

170. Warm, J. S., Parasuraman, R. & Matthews, G. Vigilance requires hard mental work and is stressful. *Hum. Factors* **50,** 433–441 (2008).

171. Virtanen, M. *et al.* Long working hours and cognitive function the Whitehall II Study. *Am. J. Epidemiol.* **169,** 596–605 (2009).

172. Tucker, P., Folkard, S. & Others. *Working time, health and safety: A research synthesis paper.* (ILO, 2012).

173. Beham, B., Präg, P. & Drobnič, S. Who's got the balance? A study of satisfaction with the work–family balance among part-time service sector employees in five western European countries. *The International Journal of Human Resource Management* **23,** 3725–3741 (2012).

174. Bannai, A. & Tamakoshi, A. The association between long working hours and

health: a systematic review of epidemiological evidence. *Scand. J. Work Environ. Health* **40,** 5–18 (2014).

175. Virtanen, M. *et al.* Long working hours and symptoms of anxiety and depression: a 5-year follow-up of the Whitehall II study. *Psychol. Med.* **41,** 2485–2494 (2011).

176. Kivimäki, M. *et al.* Work stress, weight gain and weight loss: evidence for bidirectional effects of job strain on body mass index in the Whitehall II study. *Int. J. Obes.* **30,** 982–987 (2006).

177. Byrne, R. M. J. Mental models and counterfactual thoughts about what might have been. *Trends Cogn. Sci.* **6,** 426–431 (2002).

178. Johal, S. *TIME; Everything happens for a reason.* (2017).

179. Tedeschi, R. G. & Calhoun, L. G. 'Posttraumatic growth: Conceptual foundations and empirical evidence'. *Psychol. Inq.* **15,** 1–18 (2004).

180. Ullrich, P. M. & Lutgendorf, S. K. Journaling about stressful events: effects of cognitive processing and emotional expression. *Ann. Behav. Med.* **24,** 244–250 (2002).

181. Shakespeare-Finch, J. & Lurie-Beck, J. A meta-analytic clarification of the relationship between posttraumatic growth and symptoms of posttraumatic distress disorder. *J. Anxiety Disord.* **28,** 223–229 (2014).

182. Chittenden, E. H. & Ritchie, C. S. Work-life balancing: challenges and strategies. *J. Palliat. Med.* **14,** 870–874 (2011).

183. Shepherd-Banigan, M., Bell, J. F., Basu, A., Booth-LaForce, C. & Harris, J. R. Workplace Stress and Working from Home Influence Depressive Symptoms Among Employed Women with Young Children. *Int. J. Behav. Med.* **23,** 102–111 (2016).

184. Creswell, J. D. Mindfulness Interventions. *Annu. Rev. Psychol.* **68,** 491–516 (2017).

185. Donald, J. N., Atkins, P. W. B., Parker, P. D., Christie, A. M. & Ryan, R. M. Daily stress and the benefits of mindfulness: Examining the daily and longitudinal relations between present-moment awareness and stress responses. *J. Res. Pers.* **65,** 30–37 (2016).

186. Brown, R. P. & Gerbarg, P. L. Yoga breathing, meditation, and longevity. *Ann. N. Y. Acad. Sci.* **1172,** 54–62 (2009).

187. Singleton, O. *et al.* Change in Brainstem Gray Matter Concentration Following a Mindfulness-Based Intervention is Correlated with Improvement in Psychological Well-Being. *Front. Hum. Neurosci.* **8,** 33 (2014).

188. Garland, E. L. *et al.* Upward spirals of positive emotions counter downward spirals of negativity: insights from the broaden-and-build theory and affective neuroscience on the treatment of emotion dysfunctions and deficits in psychopathology. *Clin. Psychol. Rev.* **30,** 849–864 (2010).

189. Uusiautti, S. On the positive connection between success and happiness. *International Journal of Research Studies in Psychology* **3,** (2013).

190. Achor, S. *The Happiness Advantage: The Seven Principles of Positive Psychology that Fuel Success and Performance at Work.* (Random House, 2011).

191. Arthington, P. Mindfulness: A critical perspective. *Community Psychology in Global Perspective* **2,** 87–104 (2016).

192. McLaughlin, K. A., Borkovec, T. D. & Sibrava, N. J. The effects of worry and rumination on affect states and cognitive activity. *Behav. Ther.* **38,** 23–38 (2007).

193. Hölzel, B. K. *et al.* Neural mechanisms of symptom improvements in

generalized anxiety disorder following mindfulness training. *Neuroimage Clin* **2**, 448–458 (2013).

194. Teasdale, J. D. & Segal, Z. V. *The mindful way through depression: Freeing yourself from chronic unhappiness.* (Guilford Press, 2007).

195. Brewer, J. A., Bowen, S., Smith, J. T., Marlatt, G. A. & Potenza, M. N. Mindfulness-based treatments for co-occurring depression and substance use disorders: what can we learn from the brain? *Addiction* **105**, 1698–1706 (2010).

196. Grossman, P., Tiefenthaler-Gilmer, U., Raysz, A. & Kesper, U. Mindfulness training as an intervention for fibromyalgia: evidence of post intervention and 3-year follow-up benefits in well-being. *Psychother. Psychosom.* **76**, 226–233 (2007).

197. Carmody, J. Evolving Conceptions of Mindfulness in Clinical Settings. *J. Cogn. Psychother.* **23**, 270–280 (2009).

198. Mason, M. F. *et al.* Wandering minds: the default network and stimulus-independent thought. *Science* **315**, 393–395 (2007).

199. Farb, N. A. S. *et al.* Attending to the present: mindfulness meditation reveals distinct neural modes of self-reference. *Soc. Cogn. Affect. Neurosci.* **2**, 313–322 (2007).

200. Farb, N. A. S. *et al.* Minding one's emotions: mindfulness training alters the neural expression of sadness. *Emotion* **10**, 25–33 (2010).

201. Quirk, G. J. *et al.* Erasing fear memories with extinction training. *J. Neurosci.* **30**, 14993–14997 (2010).

202. Brown, K. W. & Ryan, R. M. Mindful Attention Awareness Scale. *Psyctests Dataset* doi:10.1037/t04259-000

203. Luo, Y., Hawkley, L. C., Waite, L. J. & Cacioppo, J. T. Loneliness, health, and mortality in old age: a national longitudinal study. *Soc. Sci. Med.* **74**, 907–914 (2012).

204. Larson, R., Mannell, R. & Zuzanek, J. Daily well-being of older adults with friends and family. *Psychol. Aging* **1**, 117–126 (1986).

205. Diener, E. & Seligman, M. E. P. Very Happy People. *Psychol. Sci.* **13**, 81–84 (2002).

206. Clark, A., Flèche, S., Layard, R., Powdthavee, N. & Ward, G. Origins of Happiness: Evidence and policy implications. *VOX CEPR's Policy Portal* (2016).

207. Maisel, N. C. & Gable, S. L. *For richer... in good times... and in health: Positive processes in relationships.* 455–462 (Oxford University Press New York, 2009).

208. Diener, E. & Seligman, M. E. P. Beyond Money: Toward an Economy of Well-Being. *Psychol. Sci. Public Interest* **5**, 1–31 (2004).

209. Iacoviello, B. M. & Charney, D. S. Psychosocial facets of resilience: implications for preventing posttrauma psychopathology. *Eur. J. Psychotraumatol.* **5**, (2014).

210. Gottman, J. & Silver, N. *The seven principles for making marriage work: A practical guide from the country's foremost relationship expert.* (Harmony, 2015).

211. Wortman, J. & Lucas, R. E. Spousal similarity in life satisfaction before and after divorce. *J. Pers. Soc. Psychol.* **110**, 625–633 (2016).

212. Donnellan, M. B., Larsen-Rife, D. & Conger, R. D. Personality, family history, and competence in early adult romantic relationships. *J. Pers. Soc. Psychol.* **88**, 562–576 (2005).

213. McNulty, J. K. Should Spouses Be Demanding Less From Marriage? A Contextual Perspective on the Implications of Interpersonal Standards. *Pers. Soc. Psychol. Bull.* **42**, 444–457 (2016).

214. Simpson, J. A. Psychological Foundations of Trust. *Curr. Dir. Psychol. Sci.* **16**,

264–268 (2007).

215. Clements, M. L., Stanley, S. M. & Markman, H. J. Before they said 'I do': Discriminating among marital outcomes over 13 years. *J. Marriage Fam. Couns.* **66,** 613–626 (2004).

216. Chapman, B. P., Fiscella, K., Kawachi, I., Duberstein, P. & Muennig, P. Emotion suppression and mortality risk over a 12-year follow-up. *J. Psychosom. Res.* **75,** 381–385 (2013).

217. Stanley, S. M., Markman, H. J. & Whitton, S. W. Communication, conflict, and commitment: insights on the foundations of relationship success from a national survey. *Fam. Process* **41,** 659–675 (2002).

218. Dimberg, U., Thunberg, M. & Elmehed, K. Unconscious facial reactions to emotional facial expressions. *Psychol. Sci.* **11,** 86–89 (2000).

219. Markman, H. J., Floyd, F. J., Stanley, S. M. & Storaasli, R. D. Prevention of marital distress: a longitudinal investigation. *J. Consult. Clin. Psychol.* **56,** 210–217 (1988).

220. Gable, S. L., Gonzaga, G. C. & Strachman, A. Will you be there for me when things go right? Supportive responses to positive event disclosures. *J. Pers. Soc. Psychol.* **91,** 904–917 (2006).

221. Fredrickson, B. L. The role of positive emotions in positive psychology. The broaden-and-build theory of positive emotions. *Am. Psychol.* **56,** 218–226 (2001).

222. Gottman, J. M. *The marriage clinic: A scientifically-based marital therapy.* (WW Norton & Company, 1999).

223. Extension, P.A Fine Balance: The Magic Ratio to a Healthy. (2008). Available at:https://www.extension.purdue.edu/extmedia/cfs-744-w.pdf. (Accessed:4th January 2017).

224. Center, P. R. Modern Marriage. *pewsocialtrends.org* (2007). Available at: http://www.pewsocialtrends.org/2007/07/18/modern-marriage/. (Accessed: 12.01.20117)

225. Arriaga, X. B., Kumashiro, M., Finkel, E. J., VanderDrift, L. E. & Luchies, L. B. Filling the void: Bolstering attachment security in committed relationships. *Soc. Psychol. Personal. Sci.* **5,** 398–406 (2014).

226. Lakey, B. & Orehek, E. Relational regulation theory: a new approach to explain the link between perceived social support and mental health. *Psychol. Rev.* **118,** 482–495 (2011).

227. Ilies, R., Wilson, K. S. & Wagner, D. T. The Spillover Of Daily Job Satisfaction Onto Employees' Family Lives: The Facilitating Role Of Work-Family Integration. *Acad. Manage. J.* **52,** 87–102 (2009).

228. Calhoun, L. G., Cann, A., Tedeschi, R. G. & McMillan, J. A correlational test of the relationship between posttraumatic growth, religion, and cognitive processing. *J. Trauma. Stress* **13,** 521–527 (2000).

229. Aron, A., Norman, C. C., Aron, E. N., McKenna, C. & Heyman, R. E. Couples' shared participation in novel and arousing activities and experienced relationship quality. *J. Pers. Soc. Psychol.* **78,** 273 (2000).

230. Owens, J. C. G. Manual For The Current Relationship Interview And Scoring System.

231. Krause, D. E. Consequences of manipulation in organizations: two studies on its effects on emotions and relationships. *Psychol. Rep.* **111,** 199–218 (2012).

232. Connell, R. W. & Others. Men, masculinities and feminism. *Social Alternatives* **16,**

7 (1997).

233. Bagozzi, R. P., Wong, N. & Yi, Y. The Role of Culture and Gender in the Relationship between Positive and Negative Affect. *Cognition and Emotion* **13**, 641–672 (1999).

234. Organization, W. H. & Others. What do we mean by 'sex' and 'gender'. *Gender, Women and Health* (2010).

235. Amad, A., Ramoz, N., Thomas, P., Jardri, R. & Gorwood, P. Genetics of borderline personality disorder: systematic review and proposal of an integrative model. *Neurosci. Biobehav. Rev.* **40**, 6–19 (2014).

236. Sansone, R. A. & Sansone, L. A. Personality disorders: a nation-based perspective on prevalence. *Innov. Clin. Neurosci.* **8**, 13–18 (2011).

237. Stiglmayr, C. E. *et al.* Aversive tension in patients with borderline personality disorder: a computer-based controlled field study. *Acta Psychiatr. Scand.* **111**, 372–379 (2005).

238. Association, A. P. & Others. *Diagnostic and statistical manual of mental disorders (DSM-5®).* (American Psychiatric Pub, 2013).

239. BPD resources. Available at: http://www.bpdresources.net/. (Accessed: 12th December 2017)

240. Madan, A. & Fowler, J. C. Consistency and coherence in treatment outcome measures for borderline personality disorder. *Borderline Personal Disord Emot Dysregul* **2**, 1 (2015).

241. Zanarini, M. C., Frankenburg, F. R., Hennen, J., Reich, D. B. & Silk, K. R. The McLean Study of Adult Development (MSAD): overview and implications of the first six years of prospective follow-up. *J. Pers. Disord.* **19**, 505–523 (2005).

242. Bateman, A. & Fonagy, P. 8-year follow-up of patients treated for borderline personality disorder: mentalization-based treatment versus treatment as usual. *Am. J. Psychiatry* **165**, 631–638 (2008).

243. Singer, T. *et al.* Empathy for pain involves the affective but not sensory components of pain. *Science* **303**, 1157–1162 (2004).

244. Shammas, M. A. Telomeres, lifestyle, cancer, and aging. *Curr. Opin. Clin. Nutr. Metab. Care* **14**, 28–34 (2011).

245. Relate, Relationships Scotland. Available at: https://www.relationships-scotland.org.uk/. (Accessed: 28th August 2017)

246. Care, M. Marriage Care. Available at: http://www.marriagecare.org.uk/. (Accessed: 28th August 2017)

247. Parkes, C. M., Benjamin, B. & Fitzgerald, R. G. Broken heart: a statistical study of increased mortality among widowers. *Br. Med. J.* **1**, 740–743 (1969).

248. Amato, P. R. The Consequences of Divorce for Adults and Children. *J. Marriage Fam. Couns.* **62**, 1269–1287 (2000).

249. Amato, P. R. & Previti, D. People's reasons for divorcing gender, social class, the life course, and adjustment. *J. Fam. Issues* **24**, 602–626 (2003).

250. Tandon, S. & Mehrotra, S. Posttraumatic Growth and Its Correlates in an Indian Setting. (2016).

251. Marcks, B. A. & Woods, D. W. A comparison of thought suppression to an acceptance-based technique in the management of personal intrusive thoughts: a controlled evaluation. *Behav. Res. Ther.* **43**, 433–445 (2005).

252. Doll, A. *et al.* Mindful attention to breath regulates emotions via increased amygdala-prefrontal cortex connectivity. *Neuroimage* **134**, 305–313 (2016).

253. Hayes, S. C., Strosahl, K. D. & Wilson, K. G. *Acceptance and commitment therapy:*

An experiential approach to behavior change. (Guilford Press, 1999).

254. Wegner, D. M., Schneider, D. J., Carter, S. R., 3rd & White, T. L. Paradoxical effects of thought suppression. *J. Pers. Soc. Psychol.* **53,** 5–13 (1987).

255. Abramowitz, J. S., Tolin, D. F. & Street, G. P. Paradoxical effects of thought suppression: a meta-analysis of controlled studies. *Clin. Psychol. Rev.* **21,** 683–703 (2001).

256. Joseph, S. *What Doesn't Kill Us Makes Us Stronger: The New Psychology of Posttraumatic Growth.* (Basic Books, 2011).

257. Saffrey, C. & Ehrenberg, M. When thinking hurts: Attachment, rumination, and post relationship adjustment. *Pers. Relatsh.* **14,** 351–368 (2007).

258. Fabiansson, E. C., Denson, T. F., Moulds, M. L., Grisham, J. R. & Schira, M. M. Don't look back in anger: neural correlates of reappraisal, analytical rumination, and angry rumination during recall of an anger-inducing autobiographical memory. *Neuroimage* **59,** 2974–2981 (2012).

259. Siegel, D. J. *The Developing Mind: How Relationships and the Brain Interact to Shape Who We Are.* (Guilford Publications, 2015).

260. Ford, J. D. & Gómez, J. M. The relationship of psychological trauma and dissociative and posttraumatic stress disorders to nonsuicidal self-injury and suicidality: a review. *J. Trauma Dissociation* **16,** 232–271 (2015).

261. Fonzo, G. A. *et al.* Early life stress and the anxious brain: evidence for a neural mechanism linking childhood emotional maltreatment to anxiety in adulthood. *Psychol. Med.* **46,** 1037–1054 (2016).

262. Fletcher, A. C., Walls, J. K., Cook, E. C., Madison, K. J. & Bridges, T. H. Parenting Style as a Moderator of Associations Between Maternal Disciplinary Strategies and Child Well-Being. *J. Fam. Issues* (2008).

263. Maccoby, E. E. Socialization in the context of the family: Parent–child interaction. in *Handbook of child psychology* (ed. {P. H. Mussen (ed) and E. M. Hetherington (vol. ed.)) 1–101 (New York: Wiley).

264. Piotrowski, J. T., Lapierre, M. A. & Linebarger, D. L. Investigating Correlates of Self-Regulation in Early Childhood with a Representative Sample of English-Speaking American Families. *J. Child Fam. Stud.* **22,** 423–436 (2013).

265. Robinson, C. C., Mandleco, B., Olsen, S. F. & Hart, C. H. Authoritative, authoritarian, and permissive parenting practices: Development of a new measure. *Psychol. Rep.* **77,** 819–830 (1995).

266. Johnson, L. E. & Kelley, H. M. Permissive Parenting Style. in *Encyclopedia of Child Behavior and Development* (eds. Goldstein, S. & Naglieri, J. A.) 1080 (Springer US, 2011).

267. Baumrind, D. The Influence of Parenting Style on Adolescent Competence and Substance Use. *J. Early Adolesc.* **11,** 56–95 (1991).

268. Dwairy, M. Parenting styles and mental health of Palestinian-Arab adolescents in Israel. *Transcult. Psychiatry* **41,** 233–252 (2004).

269. van Schaik, J. E., van Baaren, R. B., Bekkering, H. & Hunnius, S. Evidence for nonconscious behavior-copying in young children. (2013).

270. National Academies of Sciences, Engineering, and Medicine, Division of Behavioral and Social Sciences and Education, Board on Children, Youth, and Families & Committee on Supporting the Parents of Young Children. *Parenting Matters: Supporting Parents of Children Ages 0-8.* (National Academies Press (US), 2016).

271. Stein, R. E. K. Children's Health, the Nation's Wealth: Assessing and

Improving Child Health. *Ambul. Pediatr.* **5,** 131–133 (2005).
272. Cicchetti, D. Resilience under conditions of extreme stress: a multilevel perspective. *World Psychiatry* **9,** 145–154 (2010).
273. Ross, S. *We're All A Little Bit Crazy: Removing the Stigma of Mental Health.* (BookBaby, 2013).
274. Nolen-Hoeksema, S., Wolfson, A., Mumme, D. & Guskin, K. Helplessness in children of depressed and nondepressed mothers. *Dev. Psychol.* **31,** 377 (1995).
275. Spasojević, J. & Alloy, L. B. Who Becomes a Depressive Ruminator? Developmental Antecedents of Ruminative Response Style. *J. Cogn. Psychother.* **16,** 405–419 (2002).
276. Schulz, R. & Sherwood, P. R. Physical and mental health effects of family caregiving. *Am. J. Nurs.* **108,** 23–7; quiz 27 (2008).
277. Childhood origins of self-destructive behavior. *Am. J. Psychiatry* **148,** 1665–1671 (1991).
278. Niedenthal, P. M., Tangney, J. P. & Gavanski, I. 'If only I weren't' versus' If only I hadn't': Distinguishing shame and guilt in conterfactual thinking. *J. Pers. Soc. Psychol.* **67,** 585 (1994).
279. [PDF]The Challenges of Adolescence - Cherish the Child Symposium 2017.
280. Lenhart, A., Purcell, K., Smith, A. & Zickuhr, K. Social Media & Mobile Internet Use among Teens and Young Adults. Millennials. *Pew internet & American life project* (2010).
281. Bolton, R. N. *et al.* Understanding Generation Y and their use of social media: a review and research agenda. *Journal of Service Management* **24,** 245–267 (2013).
282. Mueller, D.K. Running head: Pampered children - Adler Graduate School. *Alfredadler.edu/ sites* (10.2011). Available at:alfredadler.edu/sites/default/files/Mueller%20MP202011.pdf (Accessed:04.2017).
283. Schultz, W. Neuronal Reward and Decision Signals: From Theories to Data. *Physiol. Rev.* **95,** 853–951 (2015).
284. American marketing Association. Social Media Triggers a Dopamine High. *www.ama.org* Available at: https://www.ama.org/publications/MarketingNews/Pages/feeding-the-addiction.aspx. (Accessed: 1st August 2017)
285. Hernandez, L. & Hoebel, B. G. Food reward and cocaine increase extracellular dopamine in the nucleus accumbens as measured by microdialysis. *Life Sci.* **42,** 1705–1712 (1988).
286. Banerjee, N. Neurotransmitters in alcoholism: A review of neurobiological and genetic studies. *Indian J. Hum. Genet.* **20,** 20–31 (2014).
287. Green, P., Aleva, A., Robinson, C., Berger, M. & Dracup, J. Facebook, twitter and other social media are 'brain candy'.
288. Schultz, W. Getting formal with dopamine and reward. *Neuron* **36,** 241–263 (2002).
289. Dölen, G., Darvishzadeh, A., Huang, K. W. & Malenka, R. C. Social reward requires coordinated activity of nucleus accumbens oxytocin and serotonin. *Nature* **501,** 179–184 (2013).
290. Kross, E. *et al.* Facebook use predicts declines in subjective well-being in young adults. *PLoS One* **8,** e69841 (2013).
291. Pantic, I. *et al.* Association between online social networking and depression in high school students: behavioral physiology viewpoint. *Psychiatr. Danub.* **24,** 90–

93 (2012).

292. Bessière, K., Pressman, S., Kiesler, S. & Kraut, R. Effects of internet use on health and depression: a longitudinal study. *J. Med. Internet Res.* **12,** e6 (2010).

293. Pantic, I. Online social networking and mental health. *Cyberpsychol. Behav. Soc. Netw.* **17,** 652–657 (2014).

294. Wolniczak, I. *et al.* Association between Facebook dependence and poor sleep quality: a study in a sample of undergraduate students in Peru. *PLoS One* **8,** e59087 (2013).

295. Barskova, T. & Oesterreich, R. Post-traumatic growth in people living with a serious medical condition and its relations to physical and mental health: a systematic review. *Disabil. Rehabil.* **31,** 1709–1733 (2009).

296. Tangney, J. P., Baumeister, R. F. & Boone, A. L. High self-control predicts good adjustment, less pathology, better grades, and interpersonal success. *J. Pers.* **72,** 271–324 (2004).

297. Romeo, R. D. Perspectives on stress resilience and adolescent neurobehavioral function. *Neurobiol Stress* **1,** 128–133 (2015).

298. Thomsen, D. K., Schnieber, A. & Olesen, M. H. Rumination is associated with the phenomenal characteristics of autobiographical memories and future scenarios. *Memory* **19,** 574–584 (2011).

299. Ward, A. F. & Wegner, D. M. Mind-blanking: when the mind goes away. *Front. Psychol.* **4,** 650 (2013).

300. Layous, K., Chancellor, J. & Lyubomirsky, S. Positive activities as protective factors against mental health conditions. *J. Abnorm. Psychol.* **123,** 3–12 (2014).

301. Gollwitzer, P. M. Implementation intentions: Strong effects of simple plans. *Am. Psychol.* **54,** 493 (1999).

302. Webb, T. L. & Sheeran, P. Can implementation intentions help to overcome ego-depletion? *J. Exp. Soc. Psychol.* **39,** 279–286 (2003/5).

303. Bayer, U. C., Gollwitzer, P. M. & Achtziger, A. Staying on track: Planned goal striving is protected from disruptive internal states. *J. Exp. Soc. Psychol.* **46,** 505–514 (2010/5).

304. DeHart, T., Pelham, B. W. & Tennen, H. What lies beneath: Parenting style and implicit self-esteem. *J. Exp. Soc. Psychol.* **42,** 1–17 (2006/1).

305. Duncan, L. G., Coatsworth, J. D. & Greenberg, M. T. A model of mindful parenting: implications for parent-child relationships and prevention research. *Clin. Child Fam. Psychol. Rev.* **12,** 255–270 (2009).

306. Weare, K. Evidence for the impact of mindfulness on children and young people. *The Mindfulness in Schools Project in association with Mood Disorders Centre* (2012).

307. Baker, C., Dawson, D., Thair, T. & Youngs, R. *Longitudinal study of young people in England: cohort 2.* (wave 1, Research report, November 2014, 2014).

308. Gavidia-Payne, S., Denny, B., Davis, K., Francis, A. & Jackson, M. Parental resilience: A neglected construct in resilience research. *Clin. Psychol.* **19,** 111–121 (2015).

309. Kohn, A. Five Reasons to Stop Saying 'Good Job'. *Young Child.* **56,** 24–30 (2001).

310. Reid, C., Gill, F., Gore, N. & Brady, S. New ways of seeing and being: Evaluating an acceptance and mindfulness group for parents of young people with intellectual disabilities who display challenging behaviour. *J. Intellect. Disabil.* **20,** 5–17 (2016).

311. Lyubomirsky, S., Kasri, F. & Zehm, K. Dysphoric Rumination Impairs Concentration on Academic Tasks. *Cognit. Ther. Res.* **27,** 309–330 (2003).

312. Leary, M. R., Adams, C. E. & Tate, E. B. Hypo-egoic self-regulation: Exercising self-control by diminishing the influence of the self. *J. Pers.* **74,** 1803–1832 (2006).

313. Leary, M. R. & Tate, E. B. The Multi-Faceted Nature of Mindfulness. *Psychol. Inq.* **18,** 251–255 (2007).

314. Waters, L., Barsky, A., Ridd, A. & Allen, K. Contemplative Education: A Systematic, Evidence-Based Review of the effect of Meditation Interventions in Schools. *Educ. Psychol. Rev.* **27,** 103–134 (2015).

315. Weare, K. Developing mindfulness with children and young people: a review of the evidence and policy context. *J. Child. Serv.* **8,** 141–153 (2013).

316. Hanson, R. *Buddha's Brain: The Practical Neuroscience of Happiness, Love, and Wisdom.* (New Harbinger Publications, 2009).

317. Pedro-Carroll, J. L. Fostering resilience in the aftermath of divorce: The Role of Evidence-Based Programs for Children. *Fam. Court Rev.* **43,** 52–64 (2005).

318. Galante, J. *et al.* A mindfulness-based intervention to increase resilience to stress in university students (the Mindful Student Study): a pragmatic randomised controlled trial. *The Lancet Public Health* **0,** (2017).

319. White, M. P., Pahl, S., Wheeler, B. W., Depledge, M. H. & Fleming, L. E. Natural environments and subjective wellbeing: Different types of exposure are associated with different aspects of wellbeing. *Health Place* **45,** 77–84 (2017).

320. Holt-Lunstad, J., Smith, T. B. & Layton, J. B. Social relationships and mortality risk: a meta-analytic review. *PLoS Med.* **7,** e1000316 (2010).

321. Steptoe, A., Deaton, A. & Stone, A. A. Subjective wellbeing, health, and ageing. *Lancet* **385,** 640–648 (2015).

322. O'Doherty, J. *et al.* Beauty in a smile: the role of medial orbitofrontal cortex in facial attractiveness. *Neuropsychologia* **41,** 147–155 (2003).

323. Torta, R., Varetto, A. & Ravizza, L. [Laughter and smiling. The gesture between social philosophy and psychobiology]. *Minerva Psichiatr.* **31,** 21–26 (1990).

324. Kim, E. S. *et al.* Optimism and Cause-Specific Mortality: A Prospective Cohort Study. *Am. J. Epidemiol.* **185,** 21–29 (2017).

325. Diener, E. & Biswas-Diener, R. Will Money Increase Subjective Well-Being? *Soc. Indic. Res.* **57,** 119–169 (2002).

326. Ward, A., Lyubomirsky, S., Sousa, L. & Nolen-Hoeksema, S. Can't quite commit: rumination and uncertainty. *Pers. Soc. Psychol. Bull.* **29,** 96–107 (2003).

327. Nolen-Hoeksema, S., Wisco, B. E. & Lyubomirsky, S. Rethinking Rumination. *Perspect. Psychol. Sci.* **3,** 400–424 (2008).

328. Parks, A. C., Della Porta, M. D., Pierce, R. S., Zilca, R. & Lyubomirsky, S. Pursuing happiness in everyday life: the characteristics and behaviors of online happiness seekers. *Emotion* **12,** 1222–1234 (2012).

329. Dusek, J. A. *et al.* Genomic counter-stress changes induced by the relaxation response. *PLoS One* **3,** e2576 (2008).

330. Fredrickson, B. L. & Losada, M. F. Positive affect and the complex dynamics of human flourishing. *Am. Psychol.* **60,** 678–686 (2005).

29255507R00121

Printed in Poland
by Amazon Fulfillment
Poland Sp. z o.o., Wrocław